Behnam Mahmoodiyeh
Soheil Etemadi
Raheleh Alimorad Zadeh

# Generalities of the ICU and Working Principles

**Behnam Mahmoodiyeh**
**Soheil Etemadi**
**Raheleh Alimorad Zadeh**

# Generalities of the ICU and Working Principles

## in the Departments, Intensive Care

**Noor Publishing**

**Imprint**

Any brand names and product names mentioned in this book are subject to trademark, brand or patent protection and are trademarks or registered trademarks of their respective holders. The use of brand names, product names, common names, trade names, product descriptions etc. even without a particular marking in this work is in no way to be construed to mean that such names may be regarded as unrestricted in respect of trademark and brand protection legislation and could thus be used by anyone.

Cover image: www.ingimage.com

Publisher:
Noor Publishing
is a trademark of
Dodo Books Indian Ocean Ltd., member of the OmniScriptum S.R.L Publishing group
str. A.Russo 15, of. 61, Chisinau-2068, Republic of Moldova Europe
Printed at: see last page
**ISBN: 978-620-3-85851-8**

# Generalities of the ICU and Working Principles in the Departments, Intensive Care


**By**

## Dr. Behnam Mahmoodiyeh

*Fellowship of Critical Care Medicine,  Assistant Professor of Anesthesiology and Critical Care, FCCM, Arak Medical University, Islamic Republic of Iran*


## Dr. Soheil Etemadi

*Professor Assistance of Anesthesia and Critical Care Medicine Department, Modares Hospital, Saveh University of Medical Sciences, Saveh, Iran*


## Raheleh Alimorad Zadeh

*MD, Geriatrician, Firoozabadi Clinical Research Development Unit (FACRDU)*

This Book is dedicated to


*My Family's*

# Content

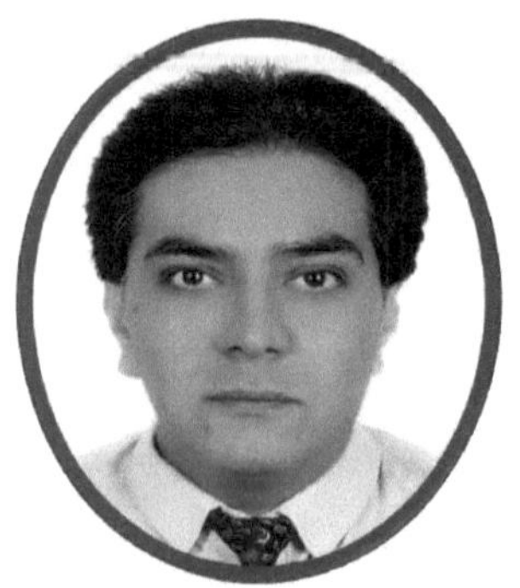

## Dr. Behnam Mahmoodiyeh

*Assistant Professor of Anesthesiology and Critical Care,
Fellowship of Critical Care Medicine, FCCM, Arak Medical
University, Islamic Republic of Iran*

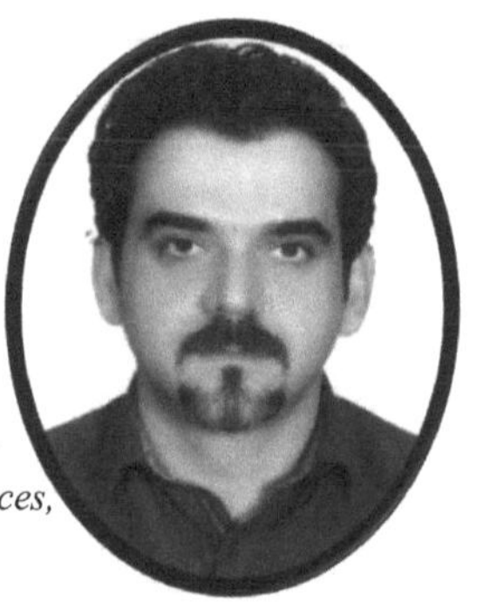

## Dr. Soheil Etemadi

*professor Assistance of Anesthesia and Critical Care Medicine
Department, Modares Hospital, Saveh University of Medical Sciences,
Saveh, Iran*

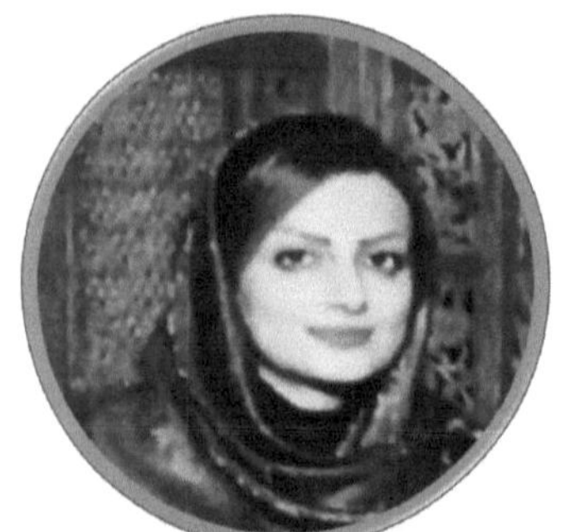

## Raheleh Alimorad Zadeh

*MD, Geriatrician, Firoozabadi Clinical Research Development
Unit (FACRDU)*

**First word**

Observance of patient rights is an essential element in promoting health care systems and patient satisfaction can be considered as one of the indicators of patient rights in the hospital. Providing high quality health care provides patients with satisfaction with medical services. Patient satisfaction is not only achieved through the use of advanced technologies, but also the behavior and performance of employees play an important role in creating patient satisfaction. Since among the health groups, the only group that has a direct and continuous relationship with the client is the nursing group, the patients' satisfaction with the hospital also depends to a large extent on their satisfaction with the nursing services; Therefore, nursing communication skills are very important in dealing with the patient

In nursing, communication between nurse and patient is the core. This relationship is of a professional type and is based on mutual trust and respect. In order to communicate to help the patient, the nursing team must be familiar with communication skills without which communication would be impossible. The nursing group communicates with patients in different ways and can convey important information to them, and because patients are in different groups in terms of belief, social, cultural and economic, therefore, a common and understandable language should be provided for both groups. There is a nurse service provider and a patient service provider, so that this connection can be made as soon as possible and can achieve the highest expected result in a short time, which is the provision of standard care and satisfaction of both groups. Also, with effective interpersonal communication, patients' needs, problems and expectations from the medical system and the disease process can be identified, and on the other hand, clients can be involved in the treatment program to accept responsibility and improve their health.

Some hospitals are equipped with special ICU-CCU wards where special patients are admitted and treated. This effect tries to provide services and ways in which the patient is resuscitated and sent back to the wards. It is hoped that it will be noticed by readers.

**Introduction**

Paying attention to the family is one of the most important pillars of patient care, because the family is often responsible for supporting the patient. Families who are unable to cope with an ICU intensive care unit may experience an emotional crisis and experience reactions of shock, anger, frustration, anxiety, and depression, especially during the first 72 hours of hospitalization. Show themselves. In some cases, they even experience more stress than patients.

The most important need of families when visiting hospitals is to ensure adequate patient care and information about the patient, prognosis and treatment process. The need for convenience has also been cited by families as the least important need. Each member of the health care team should support the patient's family members in coping with and coping with the stressful situation. Assessing the needs of the family and performing the necessary interventions to meet these needs in times of crisis is effective in reducing the anxiety of the patient's family members.

Special wards for patients are considered as stressful environments due to invasive medical and nursing procedures. Constant lighting of lamps and loud noise interfere with patients' peace of mind and sleep, and these stressors affect both their physiological and mental state. This study is a quasi-experimental study in which 5 minutes of back massage was presented to 25 patients as a stress relieving measure.

# Chapter I

*Generalities and concepts*

**The concept of intensive care**

The intensive care unit is a ward for critically ill patients with critical conditions, in which, despite various underlying diseases, there is life expectancy. In fact, the condition of patients admitted to the intensive care unit is such that they can be cared for and maintained in other wards and There are no other patients, in this ward patients are under close and constant supervision. In fact, the highest level of medical and nursing care is provided to this group of patients. It is noteworthy that the intensive care unit is equipped with the most advanced medical equipment and the medical staff selects it from among the most skilled people.

**Note:** The purpose of forming an intensive care unit is to create the conditions for the patient to be closely monitored by trained and specialized personnel. These include the following: Permanent control of vital signs such as blood pressure, respiration, heart rate, check all tests, check the patient's level of consciousness, control and adjust the devices connected to the patient (such as artificial respiration device, injection pumps) and ...

Patients are monitored momentarily and around the clock, and treatments are performed invasively and semi-invasively. Semi-invasive means direct monitoring systems such as direct measurement of intra-arterial or intracranial blood pressure and mechanical ventilation. Most prescription drugs are intensive care drugs given to patients.

In this ward, patients are monitored instantly and around the clock, and treatments are performed invasively and semi-invasively. Semi-invasive means of direct monitoring systems such as direct measurement of intra-arterial or intracranial blood pressure and induction and stimulation of endotracheal respiration by artificial respiration. Most prescription drugs are intensive care drugs given to patients. The cardiopulmonary care unit, also known as the CPU, is located in the intensive care unit.


**Types of intensive care**

The intensive care unit in each hospital is usually divided into the following types
Pediatric Intensive Care Unit (PICU)

Mobile Intensive Care Unit (MICU)

Surgical Intensive Care Unit (SICU)

Cardiopulmonary Unit Care

Neonatal Intensive Care Unit (NICU)

# TYPES OF ICU

**There are four ways of organizing an ICU.**

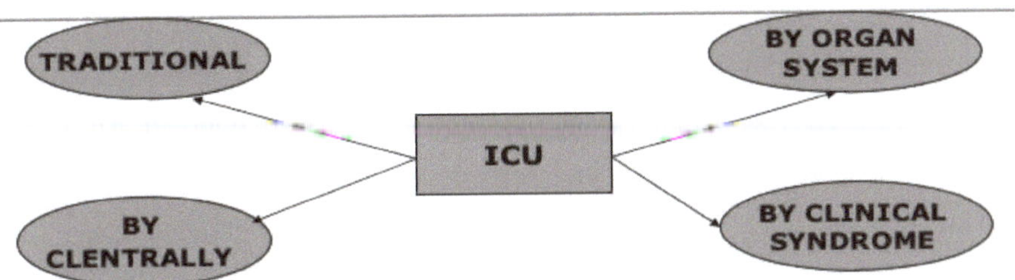


- **By Traditional Specialties:**    Surgical, Medical, Paed

- **By Organ System:**    Cardiac, Neuro, Renal, Respiratory

- **By Clinical Syndrome:**    Burn, Trauma , Stroke

4. **By Clientele:**    Neonatal, Paed., Gynae

**Figure 1.** Intensive care services

In Iran, hospital officials are required to appoint a physician working in that hospital who is envisaged in the terms of his / her specialized clinical course of intensive care (anesthesiologists, internal medicine specialists, and pulmonologists) based on capability, experience, and scientific and practical expertise. Appoint as head of the intensive care unit. If it is not possible to elect the head of the intensive care unit from the mentioned groups, the hospital director can choose one of the other specialized groups who have passed the course approved by the Ministry of Health and Medical Education and the universities as the head of the department.

The head nurse of the intensive care unit will be selected from senior nursing experts who have completed a special course called intensive care medicine. Nurses with 3 years of experience in the intensive care unit can also be selected as the second priority as the head of the intensive care unit and the head of the ICU is an anesthesiologist.

It is the responsibility of the resident physician to evaluate patients prior to admission to the intensive care unit as a clinical examination and to include the findings in the consultation form (requested by the primary care physician).

## Intensive care and intensive care

Patients need to be admitted to the intensive care unit: The vital signs (breathing, heart rate, blood pressure, etc.) should be closely and continuously monitored. All patients who have undergone major and long surgeries such as heart surgery, respiratory system, brain, etc.

Patients who need careful examination after surgery for reasons such as: decreased level of consciousness, bleeding, drop or increase in blood pressure, respiratory problems, etc.

Patients who have suffered from critical conditions such as accident, fall, trauma and injury caused by stabbing, etc., such as severe bleeding, damage to major organs of the body such as the heart, respiratory system, brain, etc., and need careful care. Be medical and nursing.

Patients with severe infections such as sepsis. Older people who need to be monitored for vital signs due to an exacerbation of the underlying disease. Any patient who needs respiratory support with a ventilator.

The intensive care unit is a special unit for critically ill patients, who, despite having many underlying diseases, have a life expectancy. In fact, the condition of patients admitted to the intensive care unit is such that it is not possible to care for and maintain them in other wards and next to other patients. In this ward, patients are under close and constant supervision. In fact, the highest level of medical and nursing care is provided to this group of patients. It is noteworthy that the intensive care unit is equipped with the most advanced medical equipment and the medical staff selects it from among the most skilled people.

In the intensive care unit, the patient's treatment is done as a team, and depending on the type of disease, different surgeons, internal medicine, cardiology, infectious diseases, etc. cooperate in this team. He is responsible for coordination and the head of the intensive care specialist team.

The rules of these wards may seem very strict, but you should note that your patient is hospitalized in this ward due to unstable physical conditions, and to maintain the safety of the ward and the hospital, as well as to help speed up the treatment process, all the rules must be observed.

Here are some common types of special care devices used in the intensive care unit: Some patients are unable to breathe normally through the airways due to severe injuries. On the other hand, if the patient is not able to breathe with the appropriate number and depth due to the severity of the injuries, the medical staff will give him breathing with the appropriate number, rhythm and depth through a mechanical ventilator. You may have seen a small monitor over the heads of patients in the intensive care unit. The device allows the nurse and physician to closely monitor vital signs such as blood pressure, heart rate, ECG, respiration rate, and temperature through wires and connections that connect to the patient.

Note that the services of the intensive care unit are such that all necessary nursing procedures such as: treatment, health, nutrition, etc. are performed by a trained and specialized team for the patient and there is no need for the patient to be present at the patient's bedside in the ward.

Sometimes it is necessary for the patient to leave the ward to perform some procedures such as: photography, CT scan, MRI, etc. In these cases, the patient may be concerned that his or her life may be endangered. Here we need to point out that there is nothing to worry about. The patient is removed from the ward by a team consisting of a nurse, physician, and staff. When the patient leaves, all the necessary equipment such as: portable artificial respiration device, cardiac monitor device, cardio-pulmonary resuscitation device bag, etc. are with him.

After the acute condition, with the opinion of the treating physician and the intensive care physician, the patient is allowed to be transferred to the inpatient wards, and this transfer does not mean that the patient's treatment is over, but it means that the patient has passed the acute phase of the disease. And for other care needs to be treated in public wards.

As a patient in the intensive care unit, you are expected to stay calm and work with the treatment team to the fullest. Trust in God Almighty and try to convey this peace to yourself and others through prayer, mystery and need for a merciful Lord.

After the patient is transferred to the general hospital wards, your mission as a companion, nurse and caregiver begins. If you want to help your patient with treatment, first try to keep your mood in good shape.

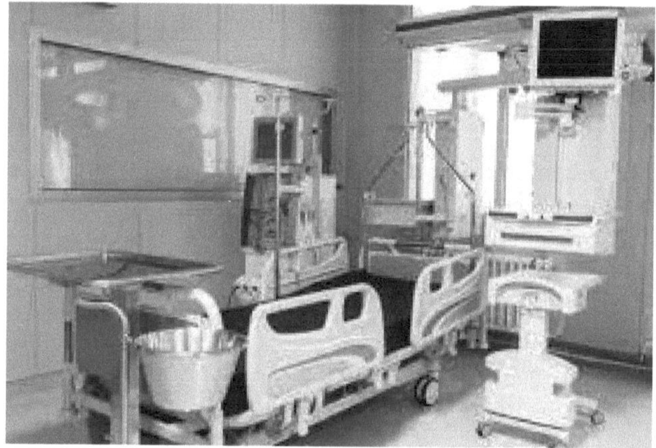

**Figure 2.** Intensive Care Unit (ICU) Expert Witnesses

**The difference between intensive care units and regular wards**

One of the differences between intensive care units and regular wards is the type of medical staff. The ICU medical staff includes people who have been trained in intensive care. The subspecialty of intensive care specializes in this department as the head of the medical staff, nurses, nutritionists and physiotherapists along with treating physicians and consultants.

The intensive care unit is usually separate for different age groups. Examples include the Neonatal Intensive Care Unit (NICU), the Child Intensive Care Unit (PICU), and the Adult Intensive Care Unit (ICU). Also, in order to further improve the physical and mental condition of people admitted to these wards, intensive care for various diseases is usually separated. Trauma ICU, internal medicine ICU, midwifery CU and heart ICU are some of these departments.

The isolation of the ICU from other parts of the hospital, the presence of advanced equipment and more experienced staff, does not mean that the condition of hospitalized patients is very serious and they are more likely to die. Rather, it means that these patients need care beyond medical and nursing care in the normal ward to return to a normal routine.

## What is an ICU?

The word ICU, which is pronounced in the Persian language ICU, is an important and caring part of hospitals. The word ICU is derived from the initials of the Latin word intensive care unit. This word in Persian means intensive care unit. The Intensive Care Unit (ICU) is a specialized unit in the hospital that provides intensive care services to patients. The intensive care unit is also known as the Intensive Therapy Unit, Intensive Treatment Unit, and Critical Care Unit. Trained medical staff such as intensive care physicians and intensive care nurses work in this department. Patients are usually admitted to the intensive care unit with life-threatening illnesses and conditions such as acute respiratory distress syndrome and infectious shock, and after major and high-risk surgeries.

## What is CCU?

The word CCU, which in Persian is called CCU, is an important part of care in medical centers. The word CCU is derived from the Latin letters of the Latin word coronary care unit, a heart attack that causes thousands of deaths every year. Myocardial infarction or myocardial infarction or heart attack is the permanent and irreversible destruction and death of a part of the heart muscle (myocardium) due to loss of blood flow and severe ischemia in that part. It happens from the heart.

This cessation of blood circulation may appear suddenly and without any previous symptoms, or it may appear after several angina attacks (chest pain). The main cause of stroke is the closure of the arteries that supply the heart. In addition to medication, open balloons and open-heart surgery (replacement of blocked arteries) are used.

Abbreviation for Cardiac Care Unit, meaning Cardiac Care Unit, for patients who have had a heart attack or are at risk for severe heart failure. CICU is also equivalent to CICU and is derived from the Cardiac Intensive Care Unit. The meaning of cardiac intensive care unit has practically the same meaning. Coronary is sometimes used instead of Cardiac, both of which have the same meaning.

In some more advanced and well-equipped heart centers, there is also an intermediate unit where the patient is taken from the CCU to the general heart ward to be better prepared to be taken to the general ward. This intermediate unit is called the SCCU or PCU, which are derived from the Subacute Coronary Care Unit and the Progressive Coronary Care Unit, respectively, and both have virtually the same meaning. This is a ward that provides intensive care to patients or the injured; Of course, the operated patients are also transferred to the I.C.U after recovery and then transferred to the ward with the doctor's order.


**Cardiac Care Unit or C.C.U**

Because the heart is a very specialized and sensitive organ and needs very special care, there is a section dedicated to cardiac care, which is the C.C.U., which is the I.C.U of the heart. The intensive care unit is a specialized unit in hospitals that provide intensive care and treatment services. This ward is also called ICU, ICU and ITU. Patients are monitored (cared for) day and night and treatments are performed invasively and semi-invasively. Semi-invasive means of direct monitoring systems, such as direct measurement of intra-arterial or intracranial blood pressure and induction and stimulation of endotracheal respiration by artificial respiration. Most prescription drugs are intensive care drugs given to patients.


**What is unstable angina?**

Unstable angina; It is a type of angina that has abnormal conditions, it is very difficult to distinguish unstable angina from unspecified infarction on Q wave. In general, it can be said; Chest pain can occur without a prelude, and stable angina, which can be felt even at rest, is unstable.

Arrhythmia or arrhythmia an arrhythmia is an abnormal heart rhythm that may be just a temporary pause and is so short that it does not affect the overall heart rate or may instead cause the heart to beat faster. Very fast or very slow, some arrhythmias do not cause any symptoms. Other arrhythmias may cause symptoms such as lightheadedness or dizziness. There are two main types of arrhythmias: Bradycardia occurs when the heart rate is very slow (less than 60 beats per minute). Tachycardia also occurs when the heart rate is very fast (more than 100 beats per minute).


## CCU feature

The main feature of the CT scan is the availability of telemetry or continuous monitoring of heart rhythm by electrocardiography. This allows for early intervention with medication or heart shock and improves the prognosis of the disease.

Patients with arrhythmias, patients with a heart attack (myocardial infarction), or unstable angina (first-time or more severe myocardial infarction) are usually admitted to CCC.

Other reasons for hospitalization in CCC include atrial fibrillation, a specific heart rhythm disorder that will usually require hospitalization, and other conditions, such as cardiac arrest in CCC, are standard treatment. Sciatica emerged in the 1960s when it became clear that careful monitoring of patients by specially trained staff, cardiovascular resuscitation, and medical procedures could reduce mortality from cardiovascular disease.

The first description of Cicio was made in 1961 by Dr. Desmond Julian of the British Chest Society, who later founded Cicio at the Royal Clinic in Edinburgh in 1964.


## Conditions of patients in the CCU

It is important to note that patients admitted to the CCU are monitored. The possibility of meeting the patient is very limited for companions in this ward, this restriction is because it jeopardizes any excitement or anxiety of the patient. Caregivers should also note that patients admitted to the CCU often do not require any accompaniment. The medical staff of this department is responsible for nutrition, health issues and treatment of the patient. The most important task for the patient is to keep calm and calm. Companions admitted to the CCU ward should understand the conditions of this ward and work with the medical staff to improve their patient. They should try to avoid making untimely appointments or repeated calls. The duty of the staff of this ward is to take care of the patient and complete the treatment measures. In case of wrong behaviors of the companions, the patient's treatment plan will be disrupted, and the visit time of the patient will be tried as short as possible. The visit should also be done with hygiene tips to prevent infection. These include the use of special gowns, shoes, masks and hand sanitizers.

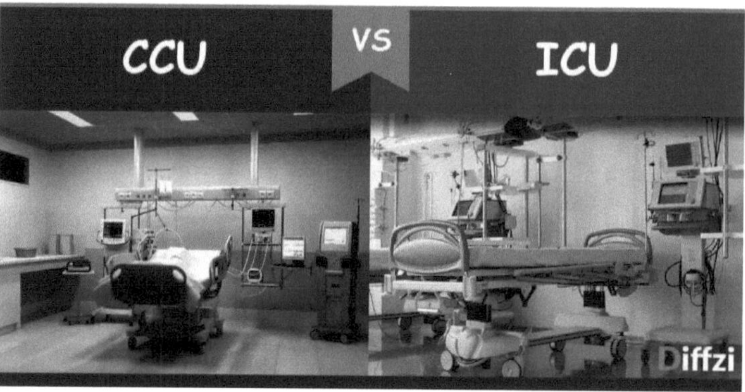


**Figure 3.** CCU vs. ICU in a Hospital

## Common equipment in these sections

Common equipment available in ICUs, including mechanical ventilators to help patients breathe through the trachea, heart rate monitors including telemetry equipment, external pacemakers, and dialysis equipment for problems. Kidney, equipment for continuous monitoring of bodily functions, network of intravenous tubes, feeding tubes, nasogastric tubes (nasogastric tubes), drainage or suction pumps, drains and catheters, are a set of drugs for the treatment of early hospital admission complications.

The main focus of ICU personnel is patients with insufficiency of the body's major systems, including the respiratory system, cardiovascular system, gastrointestinal tract, or other body systems. These patients usually need ongoing care in the form of medication supervision or respiratory therapies, such as those in places where decisions are made quickly and appropriate treatments are provided quickly. Many patients in the ICU usually enter the ward after surgery when they are at risk for side effects or traumatic surgery. The equipment of the intensive care unit for the patient's family members can be scary.

The list of ICU equipment includes heart monitors, blood pressure monitors, heart rate monitors, ventilators, fluid drainage devices both inside and outside the patient, and other equipment to control various body functions. No matter what abnormality the patient has, the ICU equipment helps the staff to control the patient's immediate condition. The pediatric ICU has the same general ICU equipment, except that the size of some pediatric intensive care equipment should be considered.

The quality of the equipment available in the intensive care unit is related to the quality of nursing and the clinical competence of the medical staff. The safety, efficiency, and cost of providing medical care to patients without the necessary equipment and proper environmental design will certainly be reduced. In determining what equipment should be in the ICU room, the whole performance plan should be considered, especially planning factors such as the type of patient care, patient equipment, and the size of the ward.

The quality of care provided in the ICU requires a variety of monitoring equipment. Patients in the ICU are usually connected to multiple wires of different monitoring devices. When detected scales are acceptable, monitors alert care team members with warnings.

Repeated warnings from these monitors can be frightening for the patient and his family. It is best to keep in mind that these highly advanced devices are designed to provide the best possible care. A list of some of the ICU room monitoring equipment includes:

**Cardiac or heart monitors**

These devices are used to control the electrical activity of the heart. These tools are similar to a computer screen and show the movement of traces along the screen. Cardiac monitors have electrodes that are attached to the patient's chest by adhesive pads.

**• Pulse oximeter**

This device enables the medical team to control the oxygen saturation in the blood. The pulse oximeter is similar to a clothespin and attaches to the patient's finger or is very small and attaches to the eardrum. This device creates short-wavelength infrared waves and receives long-wavelength waves and measures the oxygen saturation of arterial blood. The presence of shivering or some nail colors interferes with the absorption of waves.

**• Swan Gonz catheter**

A pulmonary artery catheter is used to measure the amount of fluid that has accumulated in the heart, as well as how the heart works. It enters the body through the large arteries of the neck or chest and travels in a tortuous direction toward the heart.

**• Arterial line or arterial line**

This device, also known as an arterial catheter, is used to monitor blood pressure continuously. An arterial catheter is usually inserted into the arteries of the wrist and sometimes into the curvature of the elbow (the brachial artery should not be) or the groin. This instrument creates a rejection or oscillation on the monitor that is similar to the lines created on the heart monitor but with a different wave. Arthraline may also be used to draw blood. It is mainly used for the radial and ulnar arteries in the hand or the femoral artery of the thigh.

**Mechanical ventilation**

Patients with severe acute respiratory infection may need supplemental oxygen and mechanical respiratory support. High Flow Nasal Cannula for Respiratory Support in Adult Patients Admitted to the High Flow Nasal Cannulae Intensive Care Unit (HFNC) directs high airflow and oxygenated moist mixture through the wide-opening nasal cannula and may Useful in providing respiratory support for adult patients with acute respiratory failure in the intensive care unit (ICU). This review evaluates the safety and efficacy of HFNC compared to comparative interventions for treatment failure, mortality, adverse events, duration of respiratory support, length of hospital stay and ICU, respiratory effects, patient-reported outcomes, and treatment costs.

**The purpose of mechanical ventilation**

- ➢ Improve ventilation and oxygenation
- ➢ Correction of respiratory failure or respiratory effort
- ➢ Creating tolerance and comfort in the patient
- ➢ Choose the right fashion and settings based on ventilation goals
- ➢ Provide safe care by health workers to patients at risk of infection

Physical examination of the airway to diagnose difficult airway management in adult patients The seemingly natural failure of upper airway management is strongly associated with mortality and morbidity. The four indicators of difficulty in breathing are: difficulty in applying face mask ventilation, difficult laryngoscopy, difficulty in tracheal intubation, and unsuccessful intubation.

Screening tests Many hospital conditions are used in clinical practice to identify high-risk individuals who are at risk for airway problems. However, the accuracy and benefits of these experiments have not yet been determined. The purpose of this review study is to identify and compare the diagnostic accuracy of Mallampati classification and other common classifications used for airway examination tests to assess the physical condition of adult patients without obvious anatomical abnormalities.

Chronic obstructive pulmonary disease (COPD) leads to hospitalization in the intensive care unit (ICU) and the use of non-invasive mechanical ventilation (NMV) in this area reduces the need for intubation in patients with acute attacks of COPD. However, patients with COPD who fail treatment with noninvasive ventilation may require invasive mechanical ventilation (IMV). Acetazolamide has been used for decades as a respiratory stimulant for patients with COPD and metabolic alkalosis (increased alkalinity of body fluids due to increased alkaline absorption or decreased acid concentration), and no placebo-controlled trial has been performed to confirm this approach.

According to a study published in JAMA, the use of acetazolamide respiratory stimulants in patients with chronic pulmonary insufficiency (COPD) and metabolic alkalosis using mechanical ventilation does not reduce the duration of invasive mechanical ventilation (IMV). For 382 patients with COPD who were expected to require mechanical ventilation for more than 24 hours in cases of pure or mixed metabolic alkalosis, the researchers randomly injected acetazolamide (500 to 1000 mg / day) to 24 hours randomly.

Treatment was started within the first 48 hours of ICU admission and continued for a maximum of 28 days throughout the patient's ICU admission. 380 patients were included in this evaluation for the purpose of treatment (from October 2011 to July 2014, in 15 ICU wards in France). The main purpose of this study was to measure the duration of invasive mechanical ventilation through endotracheal intubation or tracheotomy. Side effects of non-invasive ventilation after removal of the fallopian tube, length of stay in the ICU and mortality in the ICU did not differ between the two groups. The researchers note that the main finding of this study (reducing the duration of aggressive mechanical ventilation) should be considered with caution. In fact, this study may show significant clinical benefits of acetazolamide for the primary endpoint, which is not statistically significant due to the potential lack of potency at the primary end point.

**Respiratory support**

Timely oxygenation and prevention of patient hypoxia, accelerating the process of improving his respiratory status, reducing the length of hospital stay, managing hospital beds and teaching all respiratory issues to medical staff

The current situation and the high number of staff with Covid and the entry of inexperienced nurses from other departments to the ICU, the impossibility of training classes due to the prevalence of coronation, the need for optimal management of oxygen delivery to patients, emphasis on intubation as much as possible and the priority of using NIV and Bipap The time-consuming and expensive ventilator training across the country, usually by medical engineers, doubles the need to form this unit / team.

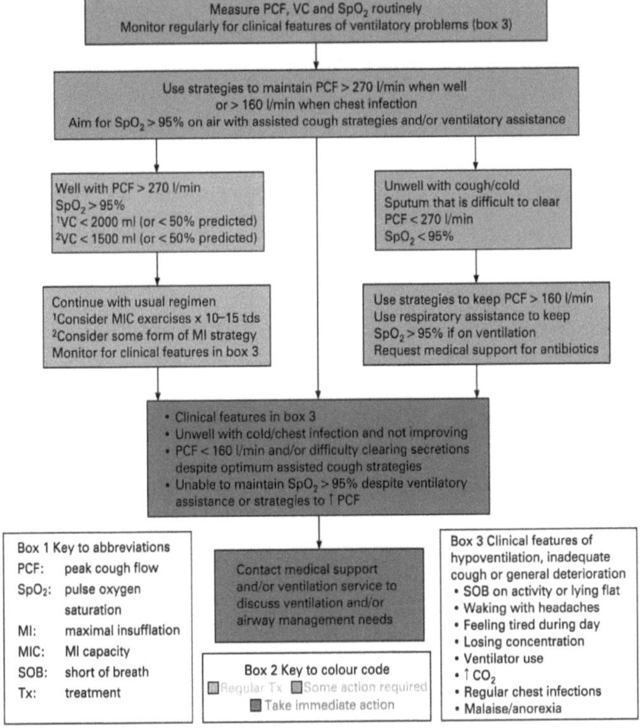


**Figure 4.** Guidelines for the physiotherapy management of the adult, medical, spontaneously

**Respiratory Support Team Tasks**

- ➢ Adjusting and monitoring the performance of Bipap devices and ventilators, according to the ABG of patients and changes) if necessary (in the settings of the device with coordination of lung / internal / anesthesia in intubated hospital patients, especially acute patients waiting for bed ICU.

- ➢ Adjusting portable ventilator devices during the transfer of patients to imaging units for CT and MRI.

- ➢ Maintenance and care of ventilators and BIPAP devices and surplus breathing apparatus, if a separate unit / room is considered

- ➢ Continuous monitoring of the correctness and health of the operation of ventilators, BIPAP devices and nebulizers in all departments.

- ➢ Monitoring ventilator alarms and settings made by the nurse

- ➢ Participation / membership in the hospital resuscitation code group and setting the ventilator if necessary

- ➢ Holding theoretical and practical training courses for nurses, interns and residents) according to the conditions of recent days as follows:
  - ✓ CPR
  - ✓ Proper oxygen therapy for staff, especially in COPD
  - ✓ How to use incentive sprays and spirometry
  - ✓ Proper training in the use of oxygen capsules, ventilators
  - ✓ How to work with BIPAP
  - ✓ ABG interpretation
  - ✓ How to work with DC shock
  - ✓ Nursing care for intubation and tracheostomy patients
  - ✓ Monitoring patient safety in preventing VAP of intubated patients
  - ✓ How to use the home BIPAP device and teach the correct diet to patients discharged with the device and file for these patients by recording the device settings and VBG

➤ Evaluation of patients' clinical condition in ICU and other wards, in order to extubate patients under the supervision of the treating physician as soon as possible

➤ Cooperation with physicians in diagnosis and treatment of the disease

➤ Performing sleep tests from patients (according to the relationship between the need for a BIPAP device and sleep tests

**Respiratory resuscitation maneuver**

Resuscitation maneuvers for adults with acute respiratory distress syndrome using mechanical ventilation. Resuscitation maneuvers include a temporary increase in airway pressure applied when using a mechanical ventilation device to open (resuscitate) collapsed parts of the lung and increase the number of respiratory alveoli participating in t volume. The amount of air inhaled and exhaled) is the ventilation device. Resuscitation maneuvers are often used to treat patients in the intensive care unit with acute respiratory distress syndrome (ARDS), but the effects of these treatments and clinical outcomes are not well understood. The aim of this review study was to determine the effects of resuscitation maneuvers on mortality and mortality in adults with acute respiratory distress syndrome as well as the effects of resuscitation maneuvers on oxygenation and side effects (such as barotrauma rate).

CCA for Half-Sleep versus Back-to-Back Situation for Prevention of Ventilator-Related Pneumonia in Adults Requiring Mechanical Ventilation-Related Pneumonia (VAP) with Increased Mortality, Long-Term Hospitalization, and Increased Medical Care Costs in Clinically Ill Patients have been. The guidelines recommend a semi-sleeping position (30 ° to 45 °) to prevent VAP among patients requiring mechanical ventilation. However, due to the methodological limitations of the existing systematic review studies and the advantages and disadvantages of the semi-supine position to prevent VAP, uncertainty remains. This review study evaluates the efficacy and safety of the supine position versus the supine position to prevent ventilator-associated pneumonia (VAP) in adults in need of mechanical ventilation. Relevant CCA Comparison of Respiratory Pressure-Controlled Respiratory Pressure with Controlled

Volume for Acute Respiratory Failure Due to Acute Pulmonary Injury (ALI) or Acute Respiratory Distress Syndrome (ARDS) Acute Pulmonary Injury (ALI) and Acute Respiratory Distress Syndrome (ARDS) Acute respiratory fractures in patients are in the intensive care unit (ICU).

Mechanical ventilation of people with ALI / ARDS gives the lungs time to heal, but the respiratory system is invasive and can lead to lung damage. It is not yet known whether respiratory-related injuries are reduced if the pressure induced by the ventilator is controlled per breath or the volume of air entering each breath is limited. In this review study, controlled pressure breathing was compared with volume-controlled breathing in adults with ALI / ARDS to determine whether controlled pressure breathing reduced hospital mortality in intubated and ventilated adults.

High and low positive expiratory end pressure (PEEP) levels for adult patients with mechanical ventilation with acute lung injury and acute respiratory distress syndrome Mortality in patients with acute pulmonary injury (ALI) and acute respiratory distress syndrome (ARDS) remains high. These patients require mechanical ventilation, but this has been associated with lung damage from the respiratory tract. High levels of positive end-expiratory pressure (PEEP) can reduce this condition and improve patient survival. This review evaluates the benefits and harms of high and low PEEP levels in patients with ALI and ARDS.


**Oxygen therapy**

Oxygen as a drug has a certain amount of consumption, specific method of consumption and its own side effects. Complications of excessive oxygen consumption include:

> **Pulmonary oxygen poisoning:** Exposure of respiratory and retinal tissues to high oxygen pressure can lead to pathological changes in their tissues. The first signs of oxygen poisoning are due to its irritating effects, which appear as acute tracheobronchitis. After a few hours of oxygen respiration, 100% of the muco-ciliary activity of the airways is damaged and mucus clearance is impaired. During 6 hours after oxygen administration

✓ 100% cough without sputum, pain under the sternum and nasal congestion develops and symptoms such as fatigue, nausea, anorexia and headache may be reported. These changes are reversible if oxygen is cut off. Continued high-pressure oxygen administration may lead to changes in the lungs that mimic ARDS acute respiratory distress syndrome. Rupture of the endothelial layer of the pulmonary circulatory system leads to leakage of protein-containing fluid and leakage of fluid and white blood cells into the lungs. Cell damage can lead to cell death. The function of pulmonary macrophages is reduced and can increase the susceptibility to infection. In general, tissue damage in the lungs is caused by the production of biochemical active substances and free oxygen radicals. Discontinuation of toxic oxygen allows cells to repair, although the repair process may eventually lead to varying degrees of pulmonary fibrosis. The key to preventing lung damage from high oxygen pressure is to avoid high oxygen concentrations for long periods of time.

➤ **Absorption atelectasis**

Absorption atelectasis occurs when the alveoli collapse and gas inside the alveoli is absorbed into the bloodstream. Nitrogen is a relatively insoluble gas that naturally remains as a residual volume inside the alveoli. During respiration of high concentrations of oxygen, nitrogen may be replaced by oxygen or washed out of the alveoli. In these cases, by absorbing oxygen into the alveoli, because there is no nitrogen as a volume in the alveoli, the alveoli collapse completely or partially.

➤ **Hypoventilation and carbon dioxide narcosis**

Usually, the main stimulus is the $CO_2$ respiration center. Patients with chronic $PCO_2$ above 45 mm Hg have reduced respiratory center sensitivity to increased $CO_2$, and the respiratory center responds to reduced $PO_2$ (hypoxia) more than high $PCO_2$. Therefore, administering oxygen to these patients may cause suppression of the respiratory center, hypovontilization, hypercapnia, respiratory acidosis, loss of consciousness, and eventually apnea.

Oxygen can cause eye problems. These effects are caused by direct eye contact with high concentrations and intensities of oxygen flow. Ocular side effects include tearing, edema, visual disturbances, retinal injuries, or even retinal detachment and blindness in premature infants.

Gaseous oxygen is flammable and although it does not ignite spontaneously, it can easily catch fire if it comes in contact with a flame or spark from an electrical device.

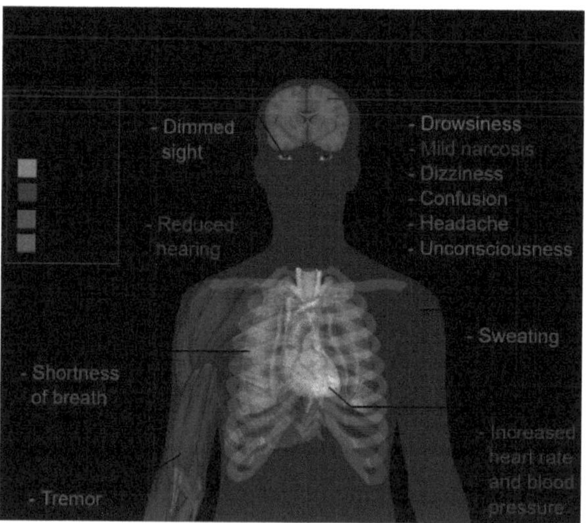


**Figure 5.** Hypercapnia

> **Causes of hypoxemia**

There are three steps to taking oxygen from the air we breathe and using it in cellular metabolism in the body:

Breathing oxygen enters the alveoli and from there into the pulmonary capillaries

Transfer of oxygen from the pulmonary arteries to the tissues

Oxygen consumption by tissues

For the health of the human body, we must make sure that all these steps are done correctly and that the cells of the body can use oxygen well.

**Some of the causes of hypoxia are**

I. **Ambient oxygen deficiency:** such as those who are at high altitudes, those who are in the smoke from a fire, and even simpler than those who are consuming oxygen in the hospital, but suddenly the central oxygen pressure drops.

II. **Hypoventilation:** This condition is seen in people in whom the number and volume of respiration is reduced due to drugs, narcotics, brain accidents or the like, and as a result, not enough oxygen reaches the alveoli and from there to the blood. Note that a patient who has received a sedative for any reason due to hypoventilation cannot defend himself against hypoxemia and his number and volume of respiration is not enough. Therefore, be careful in using sedatives and muscle relaxants in patients who are not under ventilators. Also, in patients under ventilator who receive sedatives and / or muscle relaxants, by checking the blood gas frequently, we can be sure of the appropriate set-up of the device for that patient, especially because the patient's breathing is in our hands and the device in this condition. Does not have its own.

III. **Inadequate ventilation and circulation mismatch Perfusion / Ventilation:** The third and most common cause of hypoxemia. Various lung diseases, especially viral and bacterial pneumonias, asthma, COPD, pleural effusion, etc., cause hypoxemia. Mismatch Perfusion / Ventilation hypoxemia is usually controlled with oxygen consumption.

IV. **Vascular shunt:** The fourth cause of hypoxemia. In this case, some of the pulmonary alveoli are completely filled with fluid, exudate, or inflammatory secretions, leaving the blood in the arteries that carry venous blood to these alveoli untreated, and when it comes out with blood from healthy alveoli. When mixed, they cause a severe drop in oxygen. Due to the fullness of these alveoli, increasing oxygen consumption has no effect on increasing blood oxygen, and to increase oxygen in these cases, the PEEP fluid must be pushed into the interstitial tissue with positive PEEP pressure. Ventilation / Perfusion mismatch.

**Respiratory aids**

**Pulse oximeter:** It is a device that determines the amount of oxygen saturation by using different absorption of light by oxygenated and deoxygenated hemoglobin. Pulse oximeter is a non-invasive method of determining arterial saturation of arterial hemoglobin with oxygen, and today the determination of oxygen saturation with this device is known as the fifth case of vital signs. Pulse oximetry on the patient's bed causes the blood oxygen changes to be monitored quickly, so that the amount of oxygen consumed can be adjusted without the need for repeated ABGs.

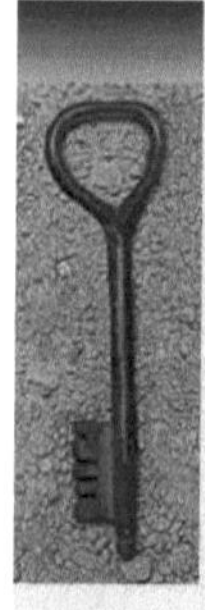



**Figure 6.** Oxygen therapy

**Oxygen with a nasal catheter:** 1 to a maximum of 6 liters per minute

If the flow of oxygen through the nasal catheter is more than 6 liters, not only the amount of $FIO_2$ received by the patient does not increase properly, but also the high flow of oxygen causes turbulence and damages the mucosa. Therefore, if the patient's oxygenation with the nasal catheter does not increase enough, another method of oxygen therapy should be used instead of raising the oxygen flow.

**Oxygen with a simple mask:** For oxygen therapy with a simple mask, the oxygen flow should be 5 to 8 liters per minute.

If an oxygen mask with a flow rate of less than 5 liters is left for the patient, the patient's exhaled $CO_2$ will not be washed out of the mask and the patient can re-inhale his exhaled $CO_2$, causing $CO_2$ retention and severe respiratory acidosis, especially in COPD patients. Therefore, the use of simple masks in COPD patients is prohibited.

## Mask with bag reservation

Masks with bag reservation are divided into two categories. If there is a gap between the bag or the storage bag and the mask and on the two holes of the mask out of the outside of the valve, the mask is called non-Rebreathing. In this case, by opening the tail, the valve between the mask and the storage bag is opened Inlet and exhale, the valve between the mask and the bag is closed and air comes out of the two outlet valves on both sides of the mask. In this case, if all these valves work properly and the mask is completely attached to the patient's face, theoretically all the patient's air is supplied from the mask and flow in the flow of oxygen and the patient actually uses 100% oxygen. If the mask does not have a valve reservation bag - Re is considered Breathing and in the best case $FIO_2$ is about 85%.

## Venture Mask

Due to the fact that in most oxygen therapy methods, changes in the volume and depth of the patient's breathing cause different volumes of room air to enter the lungs in addition to oxygen, these methods cannot create a stable and predictable $FIO_2$ for the patient. Using Bernoulli's law, in which if air is forced through a small hole, it can create negative pressure around itself and move a large, constant volume of air around it. A device called a venturi was created that could be $FIO_2$. Create a constant for the patient. Therefore, in patients with COPD or chronic hypoventilation, and high levels of oxygen can be dangerous for them, it is recommended to use a venturi mask for oxygen therapy. Venturi masks are connected to a long tube called a hose and the colored part of the venturi is placed at the connection of the hose to the oxygen tube.

On each color of the main part of the venturi is written the amount of oxygen that should be placed and the $FIO_2$ obtained from that venturi. For patients prone to $CO_2$ increase, it is best to use a 28 or 32 percent venture first, and if the $O_2Sat$ does not reach above 88, increase the venture percentage step by step. Note that the ultimate goal is to increase oxygen saturation to 88-92% and should not exceed 92% in patients with hypoventilation and / or COPD. Therefore, if the $O_2Sat$ is higher than 92, use the venturi again with a lower $FIO_2$ percentage.

## BiPAP, CPAP

If the patient is not able to provide enough oxygen, sometimes with the help of these two devices and positive pressure can help to provide oxygen to the patient. In CPAP, the device's constant positive pressure acts like PEEP, causing more alveoli to remain open at the end of exhalation. In BiPAP, positive expiratory pressure plays the role of PEEP and positive expiratory pressure plays the role of Support Pressure, causing more alveoli to remain open at the end of expiration and more external pressure during inhalation, resulting in more air entering the tail. It is very important that a person who is fully acquainted with these devices use them for the patient and adjust the set-up of the device in a way that the patient can tolerate and the patient surrenders to the device and does not deal with it. The patient's confrontation with the device can not only cause the patient to not benefit from the device, but also worsen the patient's hypoxia and hypoventilation. Some ventilators, especially newer models, can be used as Ventilation Invasive Non (NIV) and can be used instead of BiPAP and CPAP.

## Ventilator

Finally, if the patient's oxygenation cannot be maintained by non-invasive methods, or the patient's hypoventilation can be controlled, or if the patient's airway is exposed to closure, the patient should be intubated and placed under a ventilator. Remember that if you are not familiar enough with the ventilator, we can put the patient's life in serious danger. This article does not discuss all the drawbacks of using a ventilator.

**Infection control in the care unit**

With the increase in the duration of hospitalization and the cost of treatment is one of the major problems of patients admitted to hospitals, these infections with increasing mortality and complications are problematic factors in the treatment of patients, especially in neonatal intensive care units. Numerous factors such as prematurity, low weight, long hospital stay, use of antibiotics and especially the use of invasive methods such as endotracheal tube, ventricular shunt, intravascular catheter, intravenous feeding with fat emulsions in causing this infection and differences in incidence play a role. Control and prevention of nosocomial infections in the neonatal intensive care unit will not be possible without identifying the current status of these infections and their underlying factors, and numerous and different reports in different parts of the world and even in hospitals of one country regarding the status of this infection. There are. Babies in the NICU may be both a source of infection for other babies and may become infected themselves.

**Infection:** means a phenomenon in which the host is damaged due to invasion and growth and multiplication of the pathogen.

**Nosocomial infection:** An infection that occurs in a limited or diffuse manner and as a result of pathogenic reactions related to the infectious agent or its toxins in the hospital, provided that:

> At least 48-72 hours after admission to the hospital.

> At the time of admission, the person should not have obvious signs of the relevant infection and the disease should not be in its latent period.

> Have criteria related to specific infection (relevant code) to define nosocomial infection.

**Symptomatic urinary tract infection:** It is divided into three subgroups

**A) Catheter-related urinary tract infection:** The patient has a urinary catheter for more than two days and is in place at the time of catheter infection or has finally been removed the day before.

**B) Catheter-related urinary tract infection:** The patient does not have a urinary catheter and did not have it the day before the infection, or if the patient has a urinary catheter, it should not be more than 2 calendar days. The patient has at least one of the following signs or symptoms:

**C) Catheter-related or non-catheter-related urinary tract infection in infants less than one-year-old:** The patient is less than one-year-old (with or without urinary catheter), and the patient has at least one of the following signs or symptoms:

**Asymptomatic bacterial infection:** The patient with or without urinary catheter should not have any of the signs and symptoms of symptomatic urinary tract infection, i.e. lack of fever, lack of urinary incontinence, etc. In urine culture the organism is urinary with at least 10 5 microorganisms per cubic centimeter, in culture more than two types of microorganisms have not grown, a positive blood culture is exactly "similar to the organism obtained from urine culture.

**Other urinary tract infections** (including kidney, ureter, bladder, urethra, or tissue surrounding the peritoneum or space around the kidney)

> The organism is isolated from fluid culture (except urine) or tissue of the affected area.

> The patient has an abscess or has evidence of infection on anatomical examination during invasive procedures or on histopathology.

> Positive blood culture or identification of the organism in the affected area by non-culture methods

> Radiological evidence of infection (ultrasound, CT scan, MRI)

**Infection of the surgical site** (superficial infection) The infection occurred within 30 days after surgery and involved only the skin and subcutaneous tissue and has at least one of the following:

> Purulent secretion from the superficial incision site - The organism is separated from the fluid or tissue of the aseptically prepared superficial incision site.

> Superficial incision should be intentionally returned by the surgeon or treating physician or other staff member (clinical nurse or physician assistant) at least one of the painful signs or symptoms, local swelling, redness, or warmth unless the culture is negative.

> The diagnosis of superficial infection has been raised by the relevant physician.


**Surgical site infection (deep infection)**

Surgical infection (fascia and muscle layer) that occurs within 30 to 90 days depending on the surgical site with:

> Purulent discharge from the depth of the incision, provided that it is not related to another organ or space.

> Have a positive culture from the surgical site or the culture has not been performed for the patient.

> Deep infection of the surgical site that opens spontaneously or by the surgeon or when one of the following signs and symptoms, unless the wound has a negative culture.

> Temperatures above 38 ° C, local sensitivity and pain.

> Abscesses or other evidence of deep wound infection that can be seen during reoperation, histopathological or radiological examinations. Diagnosis of deep infection by the relevant doctor.

# Chapter II

*Principles of Intensive Care at CCU*

**The purpose of special care**

The recovery and health of patients admitted to intensive care units is more than anyone else in the capable and trained hands of the nurses of these units. The experience, skills and scientific support of nurses specializing in special wards are the main factor in the success of treatment protocols for these patients. Due to the increasing progress of treatment and care methods, it is necessary for the personnel of these units to be aware of the latest developments in the field of nursing and medicine. Also, virtual resources can save the time of people who want to study in this field. To achieve their goal

Patients with heart problems who need intensive care are admitted to the CCU ward. This ward is equipped with complete monitoring systems and all monitors are connected to the central monitor which is in charge of the nursing station and in front of the nurse. In each shift, one of the senior nurses is in charge of the central monitor control and coordination of ward affairs. Is in charge. For every 2 hospital beds, a trained CCU nurse is responsible for patient care and according to the conditions reflected in the control systems and the care provided by him, the necessary decisions are made and if necessary, an oncologist will be present at the patient's bedside. Patients with diagnoses of MI (myocardial infarction), stable and unstable angina, various arrhythmias, heart failure, pulmonary embolism. Myocarditis, pericarditis, deep vein thrombosis, acute pulmonary edema, pulmonary artery hypertension and valvular diseases are hospitalized in this ward.

CCU activities include:

- Intensive care of cardiovascular patients (monitoring, etc.)
- Intensive care of isolated cardiovascular patients
- Follow up the treatment of patients in other centers (dispatch for angio and ...)
- Education of cardiovascular patients (during hospitalization - after discharge)
- Hospitalization and care of patients undergoing intubation and ventilator need for ICU care until they are admitted to a better equipped hospital

**Cardiac pulse generation and electrical conduction system**

An electrical activity is necessary to produce a heartbeat as well as a system to conduct this electrical activity. Also, for adequate blood supply to body tissues, there must be a sufficient number of heartbeats, and the timing and sequence of heart muscle contractions must be carefully coordinated, so a regulatory system is needed. The natural pacemaker is the "sinus-atrial node", a microscopic group of specialized electrical cells in the heart located above the right atrium. A heartbeat occurs following an electrical stimulation by the "sinus-atrial node". This stimulus is transmitted through specific pathways to the muscle tissue cells of the heart wall. This stimulation first contracts the upper chambers of the heart, the atria, and pushes blood into the ventricles. The stimulus is then transferred to another area of the electrical cell called the atrioventricular node, which is located above the ventricles. This node acts as a delay station in the stimulation pathway and allows the atria to be completely emptied. After a short period of time, stimulation enters the ventricles through the branching pathways and leads to their contraction. Following contraction, the ventricles empty and blood enters the pulmonary artery and aorta.

Depending on the body's needs, the rate of stimulation decreases or increases. Control of the decrease or increase in heart rate is the responsibility of the sympathetic and parasympathetic nervous systems (autonomic nervous system). The autonomic nervous system is the part of the nervous system that controls the body's automatic and unconscious functions such as heart rate, blood pressure and respiration. The activity of the autonomic nervous system releases the hormones epinephrine and norepinephrine, which increase the heart rate during exercise and stress. Obtain electrical activity of the heart on ECG.


**Normal heart activity**

The number of heartbeats and the volume of blood that the heart pumps per beat depend on the health and efficiency of the heart pump. To check the health and efficiency of the heart, the heart rate is measured. Cardiac output is the amount of blood that the heart pumps into the circulatory system per minute and is obtained by multiplying the volume of blood that the left ventricle pumps per contraction (stroke volume) by the number of heart contractions per minute (heart rate) comes:

**Heart rate × heart rate = heart output**

Typically, when the body needs more blood (for example, during exercise), the going heart increases by increasing the number of heartbeats as well as by increasing the heart's contractile strength (stroke volume).

**Heart rate:** At rest, the heart rate in a healthy person is between 60 and 80 beats per minute. When activity and exercise our heart rate should increase. Age plays a decisive role in the maximum number of heartbeats allowed during exercise. The maximum number of heartbeats allowed for men during exercise for men can be calculated using the following formula:

Age - 220 = Maximum heart rate in men

For women, we multiply this number by 0.85.

Other factors that can increase your heart rate include stress and anxiety, smoking, caffeine, alcohol and some medications. Also, when a healthy person sleeps, his heart rate may drop to 40-40 beats per minute. The number of heartbeats decreases slightly with age.

**Impact volume:** Impact volume in most people is about 30 ml. A healthy heart must pump more than half (> 60%) of the blood inside each heartbeat. During exercise in non-athletes, the volume of strokes increases very slightly.

In athletes, the heart muscle is stronger and the heart cavity is larger, pumping more blood with each contraction. Athletes' hearts may increase their stroke volume by 5 times or more during exercise, so it can supply more blood to the body than non-athletes. Therefore, at rest, the number of heartbeats in athletes is lower and also the number of heartbeats in athletes' hearts increases during activity. So their heart is able to work harder and athletes can work longer without feeling tired.

**Cell anatomy of the heart**

The heart is a muscular organ located in the fibrous sac called the pericardium and is located in the chest. The narrow space between the heart and the pericardial membrane is filled with aqueous fluid that acts as a lubricant to move the heart. The walls of the heart are initially made up of myocardial cells and are called myocardium. The inner surface of the walls of the heart, which is in contact with the blood, is covered by a thin layer of cells called the endothelium, called the endocardium. This covering layer covers not only the inner surface of the heart but also the inner surface of all blood vessels.) Covers.

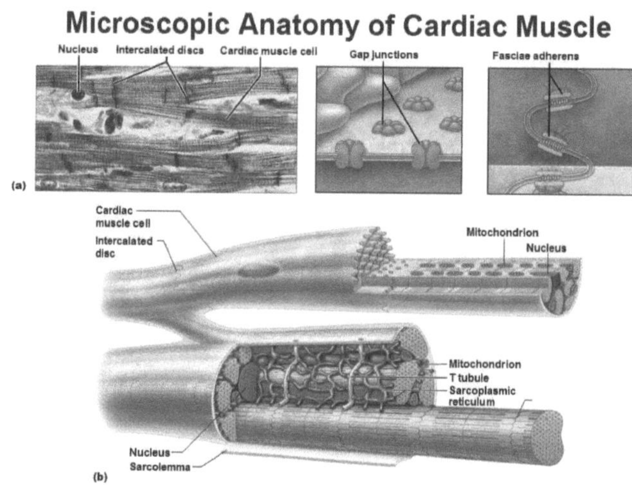


**Figure 7.** Microscopic Anatomy of Cardiac Muscle

The human heart is divided into right and left halves, each of which contains an atrium and a ventricle. Between each atrium and ventricle there is an atrioventricular valve (AV) that allows blood to flow from the atrium to the ventricle but does not allow it from the ventricle to the atrium. The AV valve on the right is called the Caspid and the left AV valve is called the mitral The opening and closing of these valves is passive due to the pressure difference between the two sides of the valves. When the blood pressure in the atrium is higher than the corresponding ventricle, the valve opens and the flow from the atrium to the ventricle is established. Conversely, when the ventricle contracts, it receives more internal pressure than the atria, and the valve between them closes tightly, so blood does not return naturally into the atria but from the right ventricle into the trunk of the pulmonary artery and into the left ventricle. The aorta is expelled.

The right ventricular duct to the pulmonary artery and the left ventricle to the aorta also have valves, called the pulmonary valve and the aortic valve, respectively. These valves are also called "crescents." These valves allow blood to flow into the arteries. They contract during ventricular contraction but prevent blood from moving in the opposite direction during ventricular rest, which act like AV valves inactivation and their opening and closing depends on the pressure difference between the two sides. Another important point about heart valves is that, when open, they provide very little resistance to current. Therefore, very small pressure differences are sufficient to establish a flow through them. In the case of disease, a valve may become so narrow that even in the case of a high resistance to blood flow. In such a case, the heart must produce an abnormally high-pressure during contraction to create flow through the valve. The openings of the superior and inferior vena cava (to the right atrium) and the openings of the pulmonary veins (to the left atrium) lack valves. However, atrial contraction pushes a small amount of blood back into the veins because atrial contraction puts pressure on and closes the veins (at the junction with the atrium), which creates a high resistance to the backflow of blood. A small amount of blood is pumped back into the veins, which causes a venous pulse to be produced in the jugular veins during atrial contraction.


**Cardiac muscle cells**

Myocardial cells are arranged in layers that are tightly connected and completely surround the cavities that are full of blood. When the walls of the cavities contract, they look like a tight fist that puts pressure on the blood inside them. The heart muscle is a combination of smooth skeletal muscle characteristics The heart muscle is striated, resembling skeletal muscle due to the arrangement of thick myosin filaments and thin actin.

However, myocardial cells are much shorter than skeletal muscle cells and have numerous branching appendages. Adjacent cells are interconnected from the end, which is called the interlocking plate (junction).

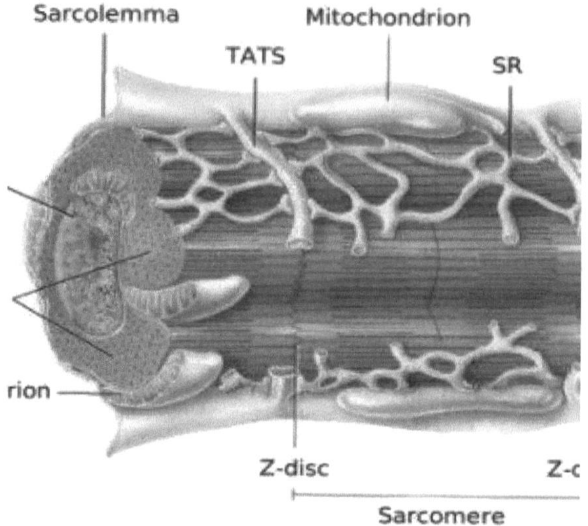



**Figure 8.** EM images of heart cell cross-sections

There are desmosomes in these plates that hold the cells together tightly, and myofibrils attach to these plates. There are junction-gaps adjacent to the intercellular plates, similar to those seen in many smooth muscles. About one percent of heart cells do not participate in the function of contraction, but have certain properties that are necessary for the normal stimulation of the heart. These cells form a network called the conduction system of the heart and communicate with other heart muscle cells through cleft junctions. The conduction system starts the heartbeat and helps the pulse to spread rapidly throughout the heart. The bottom line is about myocardial cells Certain cells in the atria secrete a family of peptide hormones called atrial natriuretic factor.

**Cardiac Nerve Innervations**

The heart receives a large number of sympathetic and parasympathetic nerve fibers, which are located in the vagus nerve. Sympathetic post angular fibers secrete primarily norepinephrine and parasympathetic acetylcholine. Norepinephrine receptors on the heart are predominantly beta-adrenergic. The hormone epinephrine secreted by the adrenal gland also binds to these receptors, and a norepinephrine-like effect is applied to the heart. Cardiac acetylcholine receptors are of the muscarinic type.

## Blood supply

Pumped blood does not exchange with myocardial cells through the cavities of the heart, food, and metabolic end products (meaning blood that contacts the walls of the heart from within). Cardiac muscle cells, like other organs, receive their blood through arteries that branch from the aorta. The blood vessels that supply the myocardium are called coronary arteries, and the blood flow through them is called coronary blood flow. The coronary arteries branch off from the very beginning of the aorta into a network of small arteries. The arterioles, capillaries, venules, and veins (like the other limbs) terminate, and most coronary veins flow into a single large vein called the coronary sinus, which drains into the right atrium.

## Coordination Heartbeat

In general, the heart is a dual pump in which the atria contract first and almost immediately after the ventricles. Myocardial muscle contraction, similar to skeletal muscle and many smooth muscles, begins with plasma membrane depolarization. As mentioned earlier, heart muscle cells are connected by cleft junctions, allowing action potentials to spread from one cell to another, so the initial stimulation of one heart cell will eventually stimulate all heart cells (hence). The heart is said to have evolved from a functional cisium age).

This initial depolarization is naturally produced by a small group of cells in the conduction system called the node sinoatrial sinus node, located in the right ten lysates near the large opening of the superior vein (superior vanacava). The action potential produced in this node then extends across the atria and ventricles and across the ventricles.

**Cardiac action potentials (cardiac action potentials)**

Like skeletal muscle cells and neurons, the resting potential of the membrane is more permeable to potassium than to sodium, and therefore the resting potential is much closer to the equilibrium potential of potassium ion (90 mV) - up to the equilibrium potential of sodium ion. One of the positive feedback is the increase in permeability to sodium, which occurs when voltage-sensitive sodium channels reopen. This is also related to membrane depolarization. (In other words, membrane depolarization causes sodium channels to open and potassium channels to close.) Again, like skeletal muscle and neurons, permeability to sodium ions is very rapid and transient. Because sodium channels close quickly.

However, unlike other irritable tissues, this condition in the heart muscle, that is, the return of sodium permeability to rest, is not associated with membrane repolarization. The membrane remains depolarized at about 0 mV in a plateau. The reasons for the continuation of this depolarization are:

- Potassium permeability is still below its resting level due to the closure of potassium channels.
- There is a significant increase in membrane permeability to calcium ions.


The second reason is more important than the two mentioned reasons, which are explained below. In myocardial cells, initial depolarization causes voltage-gated calcium channels to open in the plasma membrane, causing calcium ions to flow into the cell in the direction of their electrochemical gradient. Due to the delay in opening these channels, they are called slow channels.

The flow of calcium ions into the cell is only equivalent to the flow of positive charges of potassium out of the cell, keeping the membrane depolarized to a certain extent called the cup. Finally, repolarization occurs when the permeability of calcium and potassium returns to its original state, when the slow calcium channels are closed and the potassium channels are reopened. The action potential in atrial cells, except for SA node cells, is similar in appearance to the action potential of ventricular cells, only the duration of the duct is shorter in the atrial action potential. Conversely, there are significant differences between the action potential in most atrial and ventricular cells and the action potential in conduction system fibers. The figure for the SA node action potential shows that the resting potential of its cells is not constant but has a slow depolarization state.

**Electrocardiogram**

An electrocardiogram (ECG or K (EKG is derived from the German word kardio) is primarily a means of assessing electrical events inside the heart. The action potentials of myocardial cells can be thought of as batteries that move frequently in body fluids. These moving charges (currents) are the sum of the action potentials produced in many myocardial cells at the same time and can be detected by placing electrodes on the surface of the skin. The figure below shows a typical ECG recorded as a potential difference between the right and left wrists.

P-waves are related to currents that occur during atrial depolarization. The QRS complex occurs about 16 seconds later due to ventricular depolarization. This wave is a complex curve because the path that the ventricular depolarization wave travels through the thick walls of the ventricles varies from moment to moment, and the currents produced in body fluids change accordingly. Regardless of its shape, for example, the Q and S sections may not be present, but it is still referred to as the QRS wave.

The T wave is the result of ventricular repolarization. Atrial repolarization is not usually identified because it occurs at the same time as the QRS complex. A typical clinical ECG uses a combination of recording positions on the arms, legs, and chest to gather as much information as possible from different areas of the heart. The shape and size of the P, QRS and T waves change with the placement of the M electrodes in different situations. Again, the ECG is not a direct record of changes in membrane potential from independent myocardial cells, but a measurement of the currents produced in the extracellular fluid with changes that occur simultaneously in many cells.

Because many myocardial (heart muscle) defects alter the normal production of impasse and thus alter the shape and timing of waves, the ECG is a powerful tool for diagnosing certain types of heart disease. However, it should be emphasized that the ECG only provides information about the electrical activity of the heart. Therefore, if there is a problem with the mechanical activity of the heart but this defect does not change the electrical activity, the ECG will have no diagnostic value.

**Systole**

Through the AV node, the depolarization wave travels to the ventricles and contracts them. (QRS) Recall that just before the contraction, the aortic valve is closed and the AV valve is open. With ventricular contraction, the ventricular pressure increases rapidly, and this The pressure rapidly outputs the atrial pressure, closing the AV valve and preventing blood from returning to the atrium. Because the aortic pressure is still higher than the ventricular pressure, the aortic valve remains closed and the ventricle cannot empty This short period of isovolumic ventricular contraction ends when the rapidly rising ventricular pressure exceeds the aortic pressure, the aortic valve opens, and ventricular emptying occurs. Ventricular volume curve indicates that the discharge It is fast at first and then slows down. Note that the ventricle does not empty completely, the amount of blood that remains in the ventricle after emptying is called the systolic end volume.

In a resting adult, the stroke volume is 70 ml, the diastolic end volume is 120 ml, and the systolic end volume is 50 ml. As blood enters the aorta, the aortic pressure increases parallel to the ventricle. During discharge, there is only a very small pressure difference between the ventricle and the aorta because the aortic valve is open and offers little resistance to flow. Note that the maximum aortic and ventricular pressure is reached before the end of ventricular emptying, and that the decrease in pressure begins during the terminal part of the systole, while ventricular contraction continues. This is because the strength of the ventricular contraction and the rate of emptying blood flow decrease along the end of the systole (as shown in the ventricular volume curve) and the rate of discharge is lower than the rate of blood flow leaving the aorta. Therefore, the volume and, of course, the aortic pressure begin to decrease Diastole begins when the ventricular contraction stops and the ventricular muscle relaxes. Remember that the T-wave of the electrocardiogram is related to the end of the action potential and the beginning of ventricular repolarization. Immediately the ventricular pressure falls below the aortic pressure and the aortic valve closes, however at this time the ventricular pressure is still higher than the atrial pressure, so that the AV valve still remains closed.

This initial period of diastole (ventricular isovolometric relaxation) ends with a rapid decrease in ventricular pressure below atrial pressure, and the AV valve opens and rapid ventricular filling begins. The previous ventricular contraction presses on the elastic elements so that when the systole ends, the ventricular wall tends to turn outward. This ventricular dilation occurs much faster than when there is no elastic element, and even within the ventricle the negative pressure accelerates the production and filling of the ventricle. Therefore, some energy is stored in the myocardium during contraction, which is released during ventricular relaxation. it helps Of particular importance is the fact that ventricular filling is almost complete during the onset of diastole. This emphasizes that ventricular filling is not severely impaired during periods when the heart rate is very fast and the duration of diastole and therefore the overall filling time is reduced. However, when the heart rate reaches 200 beats per minute or more, the 50-fill time will not be enough and the volume of blood pumped will decrease during each beat. Atrial fibrillation at the beginning of diastole is an explanation for "why do not the conduction defects that eliminate the atrium as an efficient pump, (in a resting person, of course) cause severe ventricular dysfunction?" An example of this is atrial fibrillation, in which the atrium contracts in a completely diseased manner, sequentially and vibrating, and is therefore unable to function as an efficient pump. Therefore, the atrium may be conventionally considered merely as a continuation of the great veins.

**Mechanism of cardiac arrhythmias**

Cardiac arrhythmia or arrhythmia is usually caused by a malfunctioning electrical signal coordinating the heartbeat, leading to an increase or decrease in heart rate or an irregular heartbeat. Cardiac arrhythmias may be described as fluttering or palpitations that are sometimes harmless. However, some arrhythmias can be accompanied by annoying and sometimes fatal signs and symptoms. Treatment of cardiac arrhythmias often results in the control or elimination of rapid, slow, or irregular beats. In addition, since annoying arrhythmias are often exacerbated by a heart problem, they can be prevented from progressing by lifestyle changes.

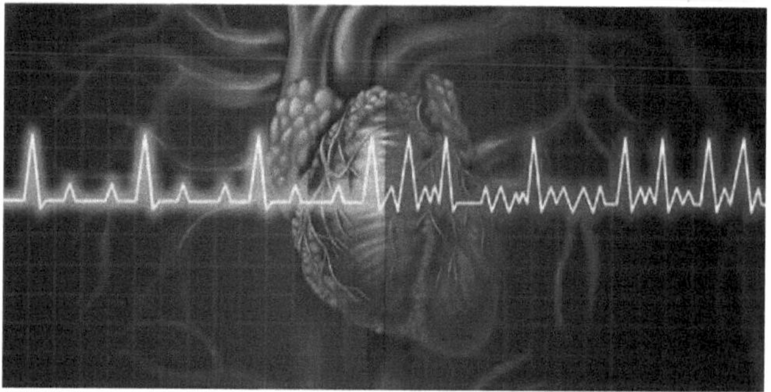

**Figure 9.** Types of cardiac arrhythmias

Doctors classify cardiac arrhythmias not only by their location but also by the change they make in the heartbeat. The types of arrhythmias are as follows:

**Tachycardia:** which means a heart rate of more than 100 beats per minute.

**Bradycardia:** which means a heart rate of less than 60 beats per minute.

Note that not all tachycardia's or bradycardias indicate heart disease. For example, during exercise, the heart rate increases to provide enough oxygen to various tissues in the body. Heart rate also decreases during sleep or complete rest.

**Causes of cardiac arrhythmia**

Certain conditions can cause cardiac arrhythmias; These conditions include the following:

- An ongoing heart attack
- Scar formation in the heart due to a heart attack
- Changes in the structure of the heart, for example due to cardiomyopathy
- Coronary heart disease (coronary artery disease)
- High blood pressure
- Hyperthyroidism (hyperthyroidism)
- Hypothyroidism (hypothyroidism)
- Diabetes
- Sleep apnea
- smoking
- Excessive alcohol or caffeine consumption
- Drug abuse
- Stress and anxiety

Some special medications and supplements such as cold medicines, anti-allergy and over-the-counter supplements

- Genetic factors
- Cardiac arrhythmia risk factors

Some conditions and diseases may increase the risk of heart arrhythmias. These conditions include the following:

- Coronary artery disease
- Heart problems and history of heart surgery
- Narrowing of the arteries of the heart
- Heart attack
- Abnormal condition of the valves
- Heart failure
- Cardiomyopathy and other heart injuries

In addition to the above, there are some other risk factors that can cause cardiac arrhythmias:

**High blood pressure:** High blood pressure increases the risk of coronary artery disease. It can also alter the transmission of electrical messages in the heart by increasing the thickness and stiffness of the ventricular walls.

**Congenital heart disease:** Having heart problems from birth can change your heart rhythm.

**Thyroid problems:** Hyperthyroidism or hypothyroidism increases the risk of arrhythmias.

**Diabetes:** Uncontrolled diabetes increases the risk of high blood pressure and coronary artery disease.

**Obstructive sleep apnea:** In this condition, the person stops breathing for a few seconds during sleep, which can cause bradycardia, atrial fibrillation and other types of arrhythmias.

**Water and Electrolyte Disorder:** Electrolytes in the blood, such as sodium, potassium, and magnesium, help produce and transmit electrical messages to the heart. Very high or very low levels of these electrolytes affect the heart's electrical messages and cause cardiac arrhythmias.


**What factors increase the risk of cardiac arrhythmia?**

**Medications and Supplements**: Some over-the-counter cough and cold medicines can cause arrhythmias.

**Excessive alcohol consumption:** Excessive alcohol consumption increases the risk of atrial fibrillation by affecting the heart's electrical messages.

**Caffeine, nicotine and drugs:** Caffeine, nicotine and other stimulants increase heart rate and cause more dangerous arrhythmias. Illegal drugs have a severe effect on the heart, causing a variety of arrhythmias and sometimes sudden death from ventricular fibrillation.


**Complications of cardiac arrhythmia**

Certain types of arrhythmias may be associated with the following complications:

**Stroke:** Cardiac arrhythmia increases the risk of blood clots. As a result of the rupture of this clot and its transfer from the heart to the brain, the blood flow of this sensitive and vital organ is disrupted and a stroke occurs. The risk of stroke increases in heart patients over the age of 65 with arrhythmias. Certain medications, such as anticoagulants, can reduce the risk of stroke or damage to other vital organs due to blood clot formation. Your doctor will consider the possibility of prescribing these drugs depending on the type of arrhythmia and the risk of blood clots.

**Heart failure:** Lack of effective pumping of blood by the heart with bradycardia or tachycardia (such as atrial fibrillation) causes long-term failure. Occasionally, heart rate control can help improve heart failure and function.


**Prevention of cardiac arrhythmias**

Having a healthy lifestyle is essential to reducing your risk of heart disease. A healthy lifestyle includes the following:

• Have a heart-healthy diet

• Regular physical activity and maintaining a normal weight

• Avoid smoking

•Quit or limit alcohol and caffeine consumption

• Reduce stress, because intense stress and anger cause cardiac arrhythmias

• Use over-the-counter medications with caution, such as cough and cold medicines, as some of these medications contain stimulants that increase heart rate.


**Treatment of cardiac arrhythmias**

Depending on the type of heart arrhythmia, different treatments may be needed. Arrhythmias usually only need treatment if they expose the person to the dangerous complications mentioned earlier.

**1) Treatment of bradycardia:** If the underlying cause of bradycardia is unknown or incurable, doctors will often use an intracardiac pacemaker to treat the problem. Because there is no suitable drug to reliably increase heart rate. The pacemaker is a small device that is usually placed near the neck. One or two wires containing the electrode come out of the pacemaker and enter the patient's heart. If the heart rate decreases or stops, the pacemaker will send stimulating electrical messages to the heart to keep it beating.

**2) Tachycardia treatment:** In the treatment of tachycardia, one of the following treatments is used:

**Vaginal nerve maneuvers:** A number of supraventricular arrhythmias can be relieved by using a series of maneuvers such as holding and breathing, dipping the head in ice water, or coughing. These maneuvers reduce the heart rate by affecting the nervous system that controls the heartbeat. However, vagal maneuvers do not respond to all types of arrhythmias.

**Use of antiarrhythmic drugs:** Many types of tachycardia are treated and the heart rate returns to normal using medication. In order to reduce the side effects of taking antiarrhythmic drugs, these drugs must be taken exactly as prescribed by your doctor. If you have atrial fibrillation, your doctor may prescribe anticoagulants to prevent clots from forming.

**Cardioversion:** Your doctor may use cardioversion if you have a specific arrhythmia, such as atrial fibrillation. Cardioversion can be done with medication or procedure. In the procedure, an electric shock is applied to the heart using pads placed in the chest. The applied electric current affects the heart's electrical messages and restores its rhythm to normal.

**Catheter burning:** In this procedure, the doctor sends one or more catheters through the arteries to the heart. The electrodes at the top of these catheters use heat, extreme cold, or radioactive energy to burn the tissue of the arrhythmic origin, thus blocking the pathway that creates it.

**3) Implantable tools:** Implantable tools may also be used in the treatment of cardiac arrhythmias. These tools include:

**Pacemaker:** A pacemaker is an implantable tool that helps control an irregular heartbeat. In this procedure, using a very small surgery, a small instrument is placed under the skin adjacent to the clavicle.

An insulating wire comes out of the pacemaker and enters the heart and stays there forever. When the pacemaker notices a normal abnormal rhythm, it sends electrical messages to the heart to stimulate it and return it to normal.

**Implantable cardioverter-defibrillator (ICD):** Physicians use this method in cases where a person is at risk for dangerous arrhythmias of the lower chambers of the heart, such as tachycardia or ventricular fibrillation.

**4) Surgery and other methods:** In some cases, surgery is the only treatment to relieve arrhythmia. Surgical procedures include:

**Maze method:** In this procedure, the surgeon cuts several points in the atria to leave a spiral tissue pattern (scar) in the heart. Because scar tissue is not able to transmit electrical messages. Therefore, it will prevent the transmission of wandering electrical messages that cause arrhythmias. This method is effective, but since it requires surgery, it is usually the last step in treatment. It is only used for people who do not respond to other treatments or for other reasons have to have heart surgery.

**Coronary artery bypass graft surgery:** If a person has severe coronary artery disease in addition to an arrhythmia, the doctor will use coronary artery bypass graft surgery. This can help improve heart blood flow.

## Atrial fibrillation

Atrial fibrillation (AF) is caused by the rapid rotation of an electrical pulse inside the atria of the heart (one of the most common arrhythmias with a reversible mechanism). And are stimulated outside the atrial sinus node. The pulse rate is about 600 beats per minute, so first we do not have regular atrial contraction, so the atria do not have the opportunity for effective contraction and are practically stationary and cannot completely drain the blood to the ventricles, so cardiac output is reduced. Second, the ventricular beats that follow the atria also become irregular and slightly inefficient. Also, stagnation of blood inside the atria (stasis) causes the formation of clots inside the atria and eventually embolism of this clot and related problems.

It is the rapid heartbeat caused by irregular electrical signals in the atrium. These messages cause rapid and uncoordinated contractions in the atrium. These electrical messages bombard the AV node, causing the ventricles to beat rapidly and irregularly. Atrial fibrillation may be transient, but in some cases it will not stop if left untreated. Atrial fibrillation is associated with dangerous complications such as stroke.


**Atrial flutter:** Atrial flutter is similar to atrial fibrillation, except that the beats in the atrial flutter are more regular than atrial fibrillation. Atrial flutter may also be associated with stroke.

**Supraventricular tachycardia:** Supraventricular tachycardia is a broad term that includes a variety of arrhythmias of higher ventricular origin, including the atria or AV nodes. These types of arrhythmias seem to cause sudden episodes of heartbeat that start and end all at once.

**Wolff-Parkinson-White Syndrome:** Wolff-Parkinson-White Syndrome is a type of supraventricular tachycardia in which there is an additional electrical pathway between the atria and the ventricles from birth. However, the person may be asymptomatic until adulthood. This extra pathway allows electrical messages to pass directly from the atrium to the ventricles without passing through the AV node, resulting in short circuits and high heart rates.


**Tachycardia in the ventricles**

Ventricular tachycardia's include:

> **Ventricular tachycardia:** Ventricular tachycardia is actually a rapid and regular heartbeat caused by abnormal electrical signals of ventricular origin. In this case, the rapid heartbeat prevents the filling and effective contraction of the ventricles to pump blood to various tissues of the body. Ventricular tachycardia in a healthy heart may not be a problem, but in heart patients it is a medical emergency and should be treated quickly.

> **Ventricular fibrillation:** Ventricular fibrillation occurs when rapid and irregular electrical signals cause the ventricle to contract rapidly and dysfunctional instead of pumping blood efficiently. This condition is very dangerous and if it does not go away within a few minutes, it will cause the death

of the patient. Most people with ventricular fibrillation usually have heart disease or severe damage.

> **Prolonged QT Syndrome:** Prolonged QT syndrome is a heart disorder that is associated with an increased risk of rapid and irregular heartbeats. In this case, the rapid beats caused by changes in the heart's electrical system may lead to a decrease in the level of consciousness and fainting that threatens a person's life. In some cases, the heart rhythm becomes so irregular that it leads to sudden death. People may be born with a genetic mutation that predisposes them to QT syndrome. In addition, some medications may cause the syndrome. Some diseases such as congenital heart defects are other causes of this syndrome.


**Bradycardia Decreased heart rate**

Although a heart rate of less than 60 beats per minute during a bradycardia rest is considered, it is usually safe. If a person is in good shape, his heart is probably able to meet the body's need for blood supply at rest at a rate of less than 60 beats per minute. In addition, a number of medications used to treat certain diseases, such as blood pressure medications, reduce heart rate. However, if the heart rate becomes so slow that it does not meet the body's needs, the person may have one of the types of bradycardia. Types of bradycardia include:

> **Patient Sinus Syndrome:** In this condition, the SA node, which is responsible for the heartbeat, does not send electrical messages properly, and the patient's heart rate changes between bradycardia and tachycardia. The patient's sinus syndrome may also be affected by Scar tissue also forms near the SA node. This is because the tissue slows down and disrupts electrical messages or blocks their transmission. Patient sinus syndrome is more common in the elderly.

> **Conductive obstruction:** Obstruction of the heart's electrical pathways can occur in or near the AV node itself, located between the atria and the ventricles. Obstruction can also occur in any part of the electrical pathways in the ventricles. Depending on the type and location of the blockage, electrical messages to the upper or lower cavities of the heart are slowed down or completely blocked. If

these messages are completely blocked, the unique cells in the AV node will be able to maintain the heartbeat, albeit more slowly than before. Some blockages may be asymptomatic, while others may cause a number of beats to rupture, resulting in bradycardia.

> Although premature heartbeat is often felt as the omission of a heartbeat. But in fact there is an extra beat in this case. You may experience an immature heartbeat from time to time, but this rarely causes a problem. However, it should be noted that an immature heartbeat can cause longer arrhythmias, especially in the elderly. Frequent premature heartbeats that last for several years can lead to heart failure. These beats may also occur at rest or as a result of stress, exercise, or exposure to stimulants such as caffeine or nicotine.

**Symptoms of cardiac arrhythmia**

Cardiac arrhythmia may be asymptomatic. In fact, your doctor may diagnose your arrhythmia during a routine checkup. However, the obvious signs and symptoms do not mean that a person is facing a serious problem. Signs and symptoms of cardiac arrhythmia include:

Feeling of fluttering of the heart in the chest

•Heartbeat (tachycardia)

• Heart slowness (bradycardia)

• Chest pain

• Shortness of breath

• Anxiety

• Fatigue

• Lightness of the head

• Sweating

• Fainting (syncope) or a state close to it

Arrhythmias may be associated with a feeling of premature heartbeat or cause the person to feel that their heart is beating too fast or too slow. Other signs and symptoms of this disease may be related to the lack of effective pumping of blood by the heart due to a very fast or very slow heartbeat. These signs and symptoms include shortness of breath, weakness, confusion, lightheadedness, fainting, or a feeling close to it, and a feeling of pain or discomfort in the chest.

## What is ventricular fibrillation?

Ventricular fibrillation is a fatal type of cardiac arrhythmia. This disorder occurs when the heart beats with rapid and irregular electrical messages. This leads to inefficient and useless contraction of the lower chambers of the heart (ie the ventricles). Without an effective beat, blood pressure drops and blood flow to vital organs is disrupted. A person with ventricular fibrillation becomes unconscious within a few seconds and then loses his or her ability to breathe. If you see this situation, it is better to call the emergency services immediately. If you do not have a trained cardiopulmonary resuscitation (CPR) person around you, use manual CPR. In this type of CPR, 100 to 120 times of uninterrupted pressure is applied to the chest every minute, and this continues until the ambulance arrives. To perform CPR, quickly press your hand on the center of the chest. This method does not require mouth-to-mouth resuscitation. If you have someone familiar with CPR around you, you can also ask them to help you breathe through your mouth. CPR can maintain the blood flow to vital organs until an electric shock occurs. Also use an external automatic defibrillator (AED). These portable defibrillators can restart the heart by delivering an electric shock.

Portable defibrillators are available in many places such as airplanes, police cars and shopping malls. They can even be made for the home. No training is required to work with this tool, the AED itself will teach you how to work and is designed to shock the person at the right time.

## Non-invasive cardioversion with heart shock

Most people are afraid of the name of electric shock to the heart, but in fact giving an electric shock to the heart is one of the safest and most often saving methods. In several cases, shock (usually 100 joules) is used for cardioversion of atrial fibrillation rhythm.

• In cases of urgent need for rapid cardioversion, such as atrial fibrillation rhythm and hypotension or cardiogenic shock, as well as refractory chest pain or acute myocardial infarction.

• In pregnant women with atrial fibrillation rhythm that is indicated for cardioversion because it is completely safe and less dangerous than drugs.

• Drug-resistant cases.

• In other cases, with the opinion of the treating physician.

Except in emergencies, cardioversion should be performed after 3 weeks of anticoagulant therapy with heparin or warfarin or, if necessary, immediate cardioversion with evidence of no left atrial clot with echocardiography (Tansesoghageal echocardiography). Continue for up to 3 weeks and sometimes a lifetime after successful diversion work.


**Surgical cardioversion (MAZ surgery):** AF surgery is performed after other heart surgeries such as valve replacement or cardiovascular bypass graft, and today, due to the possibility of ablation in less cases, heart surgery is performed only due to AF rhythm. AF surgical techniques include maze surgery, which is a very complex technique that divides the areas responsible for AF and cuts and sutures that make incisions around the pulmonary vein to connect the tissue around the pulmonary vein with the surrounding Disconnect.

In another method, simpler but less effective surgery is performed through limited thoracotomy to destroy the ganglion network. Occasionally, bipolar clamps around the pulmonary vein block triggers around the pulmonary vein. In most cases, the atrial fibrillation, where the clot forms, is also closed.


**Anatomy and physiology of respiration (Respiratory System)**

• The organs of the respiratory system are:

**Nasal cavities:** The nose is made up of two cavities separated by a wall called the septum. The nose consists of a bony cartilaginous skeleton located between the skin and the mucosa. It has many blood vessels. In the roof of the nose, there is a yellow olfactory mucosa, which includes the olfactory neurons. Are.

• Pharynx throat

• Larynx

• Trachea

• Bronchus

• Lungs

The frontal sinuses are located just above the eyebrows near the line that connects the middle septum of the nose to the frontal bone. The ethmoid sinuses are in the hypothetical line connecting the rest of the eyebrow to the nose (adjacent to the inner epicanthi of the eye) and the maxillary sinuses are below the eye and on both sides of the nose is located. The larynx is a place for breathing air to pass through and its other function is to produce sound. The largest cartilage is the thyroid cartilage, which is called the apple.

**Lungs:** The right and left lungs are the two main parts of the respiratory system. The lungs are elastic, which can help expel air from the lungs when you exhale. Each lung is surrounded by a pleura. It is located between the two lungs (Mediastinum), which contains the heart, arteries, esophagus (esophagus), trachea with its two main branches, the phrenic and vagus nerves, as well as the thoracic duct.

**Pleura:** The pleura is a thin, serous, double-layered membrane that contains a small amount of fluid that covers each of the lungs. The pressure on the lateral membrane is negative, thus preventing the lung tissue from overlapping. Rupture of the pleura causes the lungs to constrict and become paralyzed. Therefore, in order to keep the lung tissue open, the presence of the pleura is necessary to create negative pressure. The pleura consists of two layers, the visceral pleura, also known as the pulmonary pleura. The parietal pleura

The visceral and parietal pleura create a space called the pleural cavity. This cavity contains pleural fluid, the negative pressure of which keeps the lungs open. In the absence of negative pleural pressure, the elasticity of lung tissue causes the lungs to contract. The pressure between the two adjacent layers is always less than atmospheric pressure, and when inhaled, which is accompanied by an increase in chest volume, the pleural and airway pressure decreases. And air is drawn into the lungs.

The action of the tail, which allows air to enter the lungs from the atmosphere, is done through special respiratory muscles. The diaphragm muscle, which is innervated by the phrenic nerve (C3-C4-C5), is the most important respiratory muscle. This muscle is involved in the relaxed tail. The contraction of the diaphragm muscle is accompanied by a departure from the dome shape and a downward movement, and as a result, the contents of the abdomen are pushed down. Diaphragm muscle action eventually increases the volume of the chest, and due to the reduction of airway pressure relative to the atmosphere, air is transported into the lungs. The process of inhaling and exhaling is also performed with the help of external intercostal and internal intercostal muscles, so that the external intercostal muscles help the ribs that have been pulled down and forward due to the contraction of the diaphragm. Move the top and sides as well. This increases the space of the chest, which increases the volume of air entering the tail. The internal intercostal muscles, unlike the external intercostal muscles, activate the expiratory action. The ribs are the only supports for the lungs against external forces that are used to stabilize them next to the intercostal muscles. During strenuous activity, the diaphragm and intercostal muscles alone are unable to exchange large volumes of air quickly. Other muscles attached to the skeleton help raise and lower the chest. These muscles are called auxiliary breathing muscles. These muscles often do the opposite, meaning that their moving head is fixed and their fixed head moves. The sternocleidomastoid muscle, ladders, anterior teeth, large pectoralis, and small pectoralis are all attached to the thorax, sternum, and clavicle, helping to elevate the thorax. In most cases, this activity may be done by fixing the distal end of the upper limb. Some other muscles act as helpers by changing the position of the spine in the form of folding or opening and the relative change of the chest and abdomen relative to each other, for example, breathing very deeply by opening the trunk and vertebrae of the neck and contracting. The shoulders are accompanied.

The use of auxiliary muscles is not specific to the operation of the tail. For example, during the breath of fresh breath, a large amount of oxygenated air enters the lungs, this air loses oxygen and takes in carbon dioxide and must be expelled quickly from the lungs. For active breathing, the person may also be told to alternately open and close the torso for better air exchange.

## Rhythm disorders

Arrhythmia occurs when the electrical signals that coordinate the heartbeat do not reach the heart properly and do not work properly, in other words, an abnormal heart rhythm. This may be just a temporary pause, short enough not to affect the overall heart rate, or it may cause the heart to beat too fast or too slow. Some arrhythmias do not cause any symptoms. Other arrhythmias may cause symptoms such as lightheadedness or dizziness.

There are two main types of arrhythmia: Bradycardia occurs when the heart rate is very slow (less than 60 beats per minute). Tachycardia also occurs when the heart rate is very fast (more than 100 beats per minute).

## What are the symptoms of an arrhythmia?

• If the arrhythmia is short, it usually has no symptoms. It may just be in the form of missing a heartbeat that you rarely notice.

• You may feel tremors (vibrations) in your chest or neck and…

• When the arrhythmias are severe or last long enough to affect heart function, the heart may not be able to pump enough blood to the body. This can lead to feelings of tiredness or lightheadedness or lethargy. It can also lead to death.

• Tachycardia can lead to decreased ability to pump the heart, resulting in shortness of breath, chest pain, lightheadedness, decreased level of consciousness. This condition can lead to a heart attack or death if severe.

**Treatment of arrhythmias**

Before treatment, your doctor should know how an arrhythmia in your heart begins. Is this arrhythmia abnormal or not? An ECG or electrocardiogram (recording electrical messages generated by the heart on paper) is often used to diagnose arrhythmias. Other ways to check for the onset of an arrhythmia include using a portable recorder, sports stress tests, and electrophysiological tests (electrocardiography of your heart).

**Ways to treat arrhythmias include**

• Lifestyle change.

• Anticoagulants to reduce the risk of blood clots and stroke.

• Arrhythmia prevention and control drugs and treatment of related conditions such as hypertension, coronary heart disease and heart failure.

• A pacemaker that uses a battery to help regulate your heart rate.

• Cardiac defibrillation and implantable cardiac defibrillators.

• Surgery and destruction (destruction) of heart tissue.

**Hypertrophy**

Hypertrophy (from the Greek έρπέρ meaning "extra" + τροφή means "nutrition") is the increase in the volume of an organ or tissue due to the enlargement of its constituent cells.

Hypertrophy is different from hyperplasia. In hyperplasia, the cells remain about the same size, but their number increases. Although hypertrophy and hyperplasia are two distinct processes, they often occur together, such as the proliferation and growth of uterine cells during pregnancy. Which are induced by hormones.

Left ventricular hypertrophy is an enlargement and thickening of the walls of the main pumping chamber of the heart (left ventricle). What is left ventricular hypertrophy (LVH)? LVH is a term for left ventricular pumping chamber that thickens and may not work properly.

Sometimes problems such as aortic stenosis or high blood pressure can paralyze the heart muscle. In response to this excessive pressure inside the heart, the heart muscle cells may respond by thickening within the inner walls of the heart. This thick wall weakens, stiffens, and loses elasticity in the left ventricle, which can also impair healthy blood flow.

**High blood pressure:** Left ventricular hypertrophy can occur in response to certain factors such as high blood pressure or heart disease that makes the left ventricle have difficulty working. As the workload increases, the muscle tissue in the wall of the room thickens and sometimes they increase the size of their cavity.

**Heart attack and stroke:** Left ventricular hypertrophy is not controlled in people with high blood pressure, the progression of left ventricular hypertrophy puts you at risk for heart attack and stroke. Treatment of high blood pressure can help reduce your symptoms Slows and may reverse left ventricular hypertrophy.

Symptoms of hypertrophy

Left ventricular hypertrophy usually develops gradually. There may be no specific signs or symptoms, especially in the early stages of the disease.

As left ventricular hypertrophy progresses, you may experience the following symptoms:

- ✓ Shortness of breath
- ✓ Fatigue
- ✓ Chest pain, often after exercise
- ✓ Feeling of fast, trembling or throbbing heartbeat (thirst)
- ✓ Dizziness or fatigue
- ✓ Complications of left ventricular hypertrophy include:
- ✓ Decreased blood supply to the heart
- ✓ Inability of the heart to pump enough blood to the body (heart failure)
- ✓ Abnormal heart rhythm (arrhythmia)
- ✓ Unfavorable and often rapid heart rate (atrial fibrillation) that reduces blood flow to the body
- ✓ Lack of oxygen to the heart (ischemic heart disease)

✓ Stroke

✓ Sudden, unexpected beats from

# Chapter III

*Resuscitation and oxygen therapy*

## Oxygen therapy Methods

Exercise with oxygen therapy means breathing higher concentrations of oxygen during exercise. In the past, EWOT used low-current face masks or nasal cannulas that were connected to oxygen generators. Oxygen generators are devices that suck in room air, compress it, and remove argon and nitrogen.

The body is able to release oxygen with a purity of 94%, which is more than four times the natural purity of the room air. But the main devices produced only 10 liters of oxygen per minute, which took a long time to see positive results. Recent advances in EWOT have dramatically reduced the time required to view acceptable results.

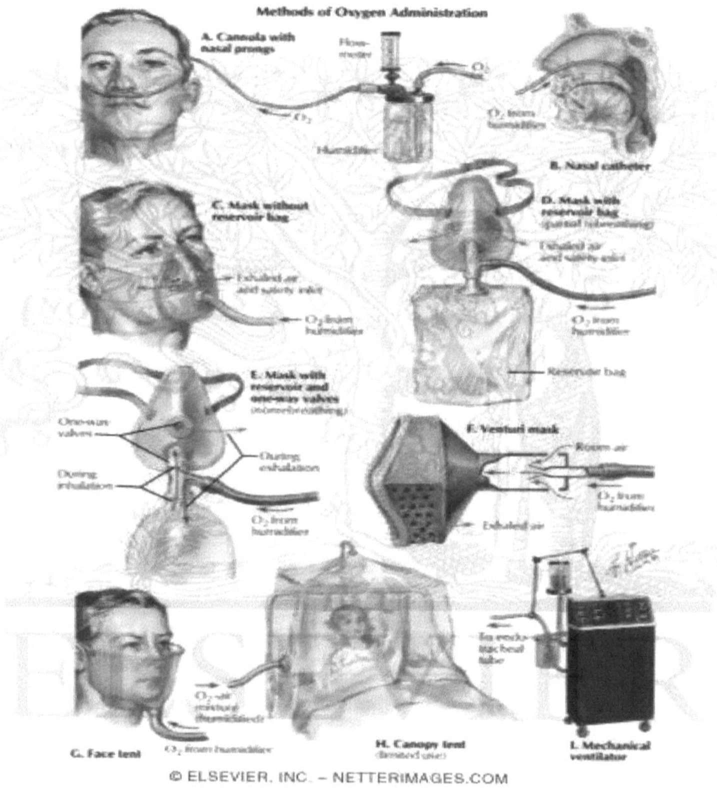


**Figure 10.** Methods of Oxygen Administration

Dr. Fan Ardennes's research suggests that a phenomenon occurs when you exercise with oxygen. This phenomenon helps reduce inflammation and swelling of microorganisms in the body. Imagine that all the pipes in your house are narrow and cannot carry enough water. Under such circumstances, one day everything will finally stop. This is exactly what happens when the body's micro vessels begin to contract; At this time, the body is unable to deliver oxygen, blood and nutrients to the organs of the body. This restriction causes pain and illness. This is where EWOT comes in and the latest technology called Maxx O2TM comes to your aid.

Breathing almost pure oxygen in such a chamber provides us with 7.5 times more oxygen than normal breathing. In one hour we can inhale 1.5 pounds (680 grams) of oxygen. Red blood cells are rapidly saturated with oxygen, but more important is the dissolution of excess oxygen in the blood plasma. Plasma, not red blood cells, play a key role. This extra oxygen helps oxygen-deficient tissues regain the oxygen they need. This action is involved in stimulating recovery, during oxygen uptake and after cessation. After oxygen is cut off, the reticuloendothelial system is activated. After hypotension, natural homeostasis maintains healthy function by stimulating adaptation to lower but normal oxygen levels.

To increase the tissue oxygen pressure by more than 50 mm Hg to induce a restorative effect, it is necessary to give the individual a small amount of almost pure oxygen with increasing pressure conditions and to increase the inlet oxygen pressure when the oxygen is at a pressure of 1.5 atmospheres. We breathe, we see. A linear increase in tissue oxygen levels at pressures 1 and 2 atmospheres can be seen in the diagram above. When the atmospheric pressure rises 100% above the normal level (2 atmospheres) the graph rises geometrically. At higher levels (more than 2 atmospheres), tissue oxygenation increases excessively (hyperoxia). Therefore, careful monitoring is needed because too much nerve sensitivity to oxygen can cause transient side effects. This sensitivity does not occur at levels less than one-third and one-fourth of the atmosphere because the body can self-regulate oxygen uptake in areas that need more oxygen and prevent oxygen from entering tissues in areas where there is enough oxygen.

Physical and transient factors sometimes produce good and varied results in different patients. The doctor cannot control the amount of oxygen that enters or leaves the patient's body, and the amount of tissue oxidative enzymes varies from patient to patient. The diagram above shows an increase in venous oxygen at different pressures. To distinguish linear increase from geometric increase, displays are marked as pressure increase and hyperbar pressure. The problem with understanding oxygen therapy is that the ambiguity between saturation and oxygen pressure is 100% versus 100 mm Hg. Only dissolved oxygen produces pressure (or partial pressure).

The difference in the amount of oxygen carried by the plasma (in solution) is caused by the difference with the oxygen of hemoglobin. One gram of hemoglobin saturates only 1.34 ml of oxygen to form oxyhemoglobin. 100 ml of a healthy person's blood at normal pressure has 19 ml of oxygen in the form of oxyhemoglobin and 0.3 ml of oxygen. Naturally, hemoglobin has a saturation of up to 98%. And the dissolved oxygen pressure is initially 95 mm Hg, which decreases to 39 mm Hg at the tissue surface. Breathing pure oxygen at 2.5 times the atmospheric pressure increases the amount of plasma dissolved oxygen by about 6 ml per 100 ml of blood. This increase in oxygen volume significantly increases the oxygen pressure and increases the oxygen pressure released at the tissue surface by up to 200 ml.

Hypertensive oxygenation helps to repair conditions in which the body is affected by low tissue oxygen levels. Multiple hyperbaric sessions help to heal a variety of conditions such as anemia, burns and compression injuries. Poor skin grafts often improve with hyperbaric oxygenation. Treatment of difficult infections with high-pressure oxygenation, including actinomycosis, osteomyelitis, diabetic wounds, gangrene, and other infections in the dead tissue, has opened up new horizons.


**Oxygen transport systems**

Jason Tebao, founder and chairman of EWOT.com, introduced the first open oxygen delivery system to the market in 2008. His EWOT products have evolved and are now based on the 15-minute fast method and scientific research by Dr. Manfred van Ardenne, author of Oxygen Babylon (a 400-page book on multi-stage oxygen therapy).

In his book, von Ardenne has researched more than 500 medical references to support the use of oxygen to improve cellular health, and provides scientific evidence based on 10,000 studies.

Oxygen is one of the most important gases in respiration, which is essential for human life. Some people with respiratory problems may not be able to get the oxygen they need. They may need extra oxygen or this treatment. Oxygen therapy in these patients increases their energy levels and sleep quality.

But there is another type of oxygen therapy that has been available to us for years and may be even more useful than oxygen therapy under pressure. Exercise combined with oxygen therapy has been a scientifically proven phenomenon that, according to research, can restore our general health back to our youth. This phenomenon is called EWOT (exercise with oxygen therapy), and is beneficial to the health of many people.

**Oxygen therapy under pressure versus EWOT**

Oxygen under pressure is a medical device that needs to be prescribed and can be a slow process. You do not exercise in pressure chambers. This means that there is no $CO_2$ production to equalize the amount of excess oxygen input. Exercise, along with oxygen therapy, works to increase your heart rate, allowing you to produce more carbon dioxide, increase relative pressure, and convert more oxygen into hypoxic tissue. Slowly This is a natural process and the optimal use of oxygen. Because EWOT increases oxygen uptake as the heart rate increases, optimal results are achieved more rapidly.

Although it certainly takes a certain amount of time and space to perform stress oxygen therapy, it does help treat conditions such as decompression, serious infections, and chronic wounds, and may even cure animal diseases. At the same time, for the average person looking to oxygenate the blood in their body - to reduce swelling, increase energy and maintain overall health - the Maxx $O_2$ is much more effective.

Exercise combined with oxygen therapy delivers oxygen to the arteries, veins, and even the smallest capillaries that make up more than 74% of your circulatory system. As oxygen circulation in the body increases, your cells receive the oxygen they need daily to process the millions of biochemical reactions they perform.

According to Dr. Van Arden, improving the flow of oxygen to the tissues of the body is very important to fight against insufficient oxygen supply, because it is a common cause of many diseases, disorders and difficulties. So why is getting enough oxygen so important? For one thing. Research has shown that hypoxia is a major cause of many cancers. According to researchers at the University of Georgia, low levels of oxygen in our cells could be the main cause of uncontrolled tumor growth in some cancers. And a study conducted at Washington State University shows that when high-pressure oxygen was used in the culture of blood cancer cells, it reduced the growth of cancer cells by up to 15 percent.

Research published in current chemistry shows that in the acute stages of cancer risk and when blood oxygen levels are very low, during hypoxemia, oxidative stress accelerates decay and gives our cells the ability to divide and grow. Lose yourself. The bottom line is that we cannot live without oxygen. And when our cells do not get enough oxygen, many aspects of our health are affected.


**Oxygen reveals blood flow**

All body processes require adequate blood flow, but stress and certain medical conditions can impair the blood's ability to release oxygen to the body's tissues. We know that depletion of oxygen in the blood can severely damage the function of the brain, liver and other organs. We need our blood to supply oxygen to all parts of the body. This is one of the main benefits of oxygen therapy. As oxygen circulation in the body increases, oxygen-rich blood can send oxygen to tissues, blood vessels, and organs.

Restoration of oxygen-rich blood flow causes capillaries to dilate. When capillaries are deficient in oxygen, they begin to swell, preventing further oxygenation. Oxygen therapy in particular (EWOT) reduces capillary swelling and improves oxygenation and blood circulation.

One of the known benefits of oxygen therapy is its ability to improve cerebral blood flow. Research shows that pressurized oxygen therapy can be used to help treat ischemic ulcers in patients with diabetes. It is hypothesized that this type of oxygen therapy is involved in the regeneration of vascular activity and affects the production of vasodilators and coronary arteries.

**Application of oxygen therapy**

This treatment is suitable for people who are not able to absorb enough oxygen. Conditions that interfere with the absorption of oxygen in the lungs are often caused by lung diseases, including:

• Asthma

• Pneumonia

• Sleep apnea

• Lung disease

• Heart failure

• Cystic fibrosis

• Respiratory damage

• Chronic obstructive pulmonary disease (COPD)

• Pulmonary bronchope dysplasia, underdeveloped lungs in infants

**Benefits of oxygen therapy**

It will also bring you the following benefits:

• Maintain safety

• Accelerate recovery after illness or injury

• Increase energy

• Improve cardiovascular health

• Supports lung / respiratory function

• Improve physical performance

• Faster recovery after exercise

• Improves vision

• Improve brain capacity / memory

• Reduce inflammation

• Help to lose weight

• Improved detoxification

**How to use oxygen therapy?**

There are several products on the market today that are used as a source of oxygen therapy. Pressure oxygen therapy is usually performed on an outpatient basis in a special chamber. To perform this type of treatment, you are placed in a container designed for one person. There are also pressurized oxygen chambers that can accommodate several people at the same time. You can also perform oxygen therapy with a nasal mask or cannula attached to an oxygen generator. The generator supplies oxygen and this oxygen is breathed through the tube. However, these types of devices have problems. The most powerful oxygen generator can produce only up to 10 liters of oxygen per minute, and we can easily breathe up to 50 liters per minute during exercise. So we need a lot more oxygen during exercise and no generator can produce that much oxygen. To solve problems with older technologies and slower impacts, Maxx $O_2$ was created that did the job in 15 minutes.

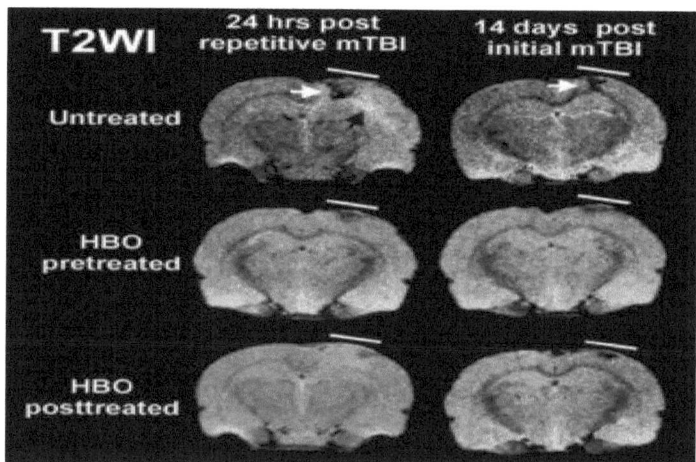


**Figure 11.** Hyperbaric oxygen therapy for traumatic brain injury

In the Maxx $O_2$, a large bag is initially filled with 900 liters of oxygen using an oxygen generator. On a full charge, the Maxx $O_2$ High Current Mask connected to a thick hose (to deliver an unlimited source of oxygen) is used to meet your needs during a 15-minute session. The generator fills the bag just before the treatment session, and when you start exercising, you only breathe in the oxygen in the bag.

You breathe out of the bag and blow $CO_2$ into the room. For more oxygen purity, pass the HEPA filter. Just one 15-minute session of Maxx $O_2$ can bring you the benefits of dozens of sessions of oxygen under pressure.


**Risks and side effects of oxygen therapy**

When EVOT is performed correctly and is not performed for more than 15 minutes in one step, there are no risks or side effects. Breathing high levels of oxygen is safe and there is no risk of oxygen toxicity. For many patients who have just started using EWOT, a sudden change in their level of physical activity can lead to side effects. For people who have not exercised for a long time and do not have enough physical endurance to endure a 15-minute session, it is better to do this procedure gradually and consult your doctor before any action.

Exercise combined with oxygen therapy is an effective way to increase oxygen circulation in the body. Unlike pressurized oxygen therapy, which involves lying in an oxygen chamber, EWOT increases your heart rate. This allows you to produce more carbon dioxide and inject more oxygen into your distal cells.


**Application of hyperbaric oxygen in brain lesions**

Ultrasound scans of the brain show that most babies with cerebral palsy have a lesion at birth. However, symptoms of muscle stiffness may not appear until months later. In cerebral palsy, the middle part of the hemispheres of the brain is damaged on one or both sides. High-risk areas in the middle part of the brain are where the control fibers of cells in the gray areas of the brain pass to the spinal cord and attach to the nerve cells in the spinal cord that function the muscles of the limbs. Lack of oxygen to the brain is referred to as hypoxia in the brain and is structural. The first brain injury from lack of oxygen is inflammation, which causes a damaging cycle that results in brain disability. Inflammation is a common finding in many brain disorders (the central nervous system, including the brain and spinal cord).

Inflammation can be directly affected by many factors including heart problems, circulatory system problems and toxic factors. Other causes of cerebral edema include infections, vitamin deficiencies, and trauma (either direct or traumatic). Problems and diseases during pregnancy include diabetes, heart disease and fetal oxygen deprivation. Inflammation of the brain, spinal cord, and hypoxia can be treated and cured over time. Swelling and hypoxia can be exacerbated by other neurological problems. Encephalitis leads to myelination of neurons (nerve cells) and vascular problems. The myelin sheath is the white tissue that covers the nerve fibers. It usually starts about a month before birth. The process of myelination begins in the spinal cord and spreads to the brain. The frontal lobe of the hemispheres of the brain is completed around the age of 22. The cerebral arteries in the uterus prepare for labor in the last 2 weeks of pregnancy. This means that if a baby is born prematurely, it will not be able to tolerate the lack of oxygen during the transfer from the mother's womb to the outside world.

This causes swelling and consequent lack of oxygen (hypoxia) in the midbrain. This incident can prevent the transfer of oligo dendrites that make myelin and direct it to the nervous system. The role of high-pressure oxygen in improving nervous system damage in infants the use of HBO, or high-pressure oxygen, greatly increases oxygen uptake in areas where fuel production is low. This is effective in reducing muscle stiffness (spasticity), increasing and improving gait, improving speech and mouthwatering.

The use of high-pressure oxygen, in areas with low metabolism, greatly increases oxygen uptake. This is effective in reducing muscle stiffness, increasing and improving gait, improving speech and mouth rinsing. The use of high pressure oxygen effectively increases and improves the released oxygen. It therefore increases the oxygen available to the tissue. It reduces inflammation and completes blood flow through the intercellular wall and blood vessels, as well as normalizes phagocytosis (poisoning) of toxic cells and clears free radicals. It also reactivates lazy cells.

**The role of high-pressure oxygen to help heal diving injuries**

Hypertensive oxygen therapy has long been used as an acceptable and well-known treatment for pressure-related diving injuries. These injuries are collectively known as hypertension disease, which includes arterial gas embolism and hypertension disease. The two diseases were described separately because their hypothetical causes were different. In fact, starting treatment and maintaining stability in an injured diver depends on the diver's condition, not on one of the two diseases DCI and AGE that the diver suffers from. Pressure relief is thought to be caused by the formation of bubbles inside tissues in which blood flow and oxygen delivery are stopped. Arterial gas embolism, on the other hand, occurs due to the entry of bubbles into the arterial bloodstream through the rupture of lung tissue.

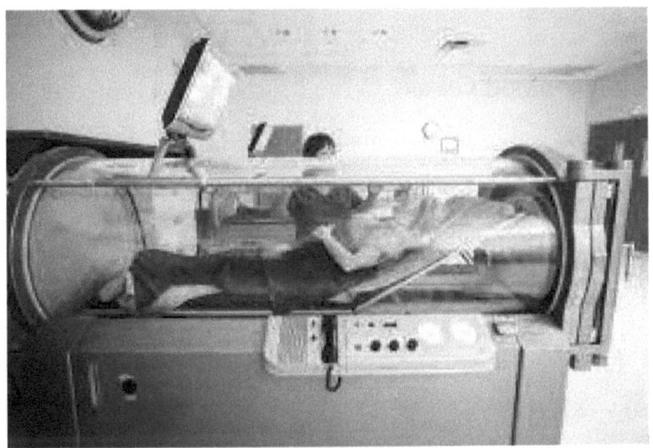

**Figure 12.** An Overview of Hyperbaric Chamber Treatment

A well-known treatment for arterial gas pressure and embolism is recurrence. Reduce the bubble size and remove it gradually.

In cases of arterial gas embolism and severe hypertensive disease, hyperbaric pressure is critical to reduce the size of large bubbles. Hyperbaric oxygen therapy begins with a special protocol called a treatment schedule. There are different treatment tables, each with its own time program of pressure as it begins to breathe oxygen. The most common treatment schedule for recreational diving accidents is Table 6 of the US Navy. Other treatment tables have been designed for different types of diving accidents with different symptoms. These divers dive to a depth of 108 feet (33 meters) or more for hours or days.

## Application of hypertensive oxygen therapy in severe headaches

Researchers have found that high-pressure oxygen therapy can stop pain during migraine attacks. Oxygen therapy with natural pressure also relieves pain in patients with cluster headaches. Migraines typically cause throbbing pain in an area of the head that is often accompanied by nausea, vomiting, or sensitivity to light and sound. Cluster headaches cause acute pain on one side of the head along with pain in the eye. It can last from 15 minutes to a few hours, and recurrent attacks occur over weeks to months, followed by asymptomatic episodes. Men are three times more likely than women to have cluster headaches.

In a migraine attack, the blood vessels in the head dilate. Hypertensive oxygen causes narrowing of the arteries, which may cause pain relief. High-pressure oxygen inhibits "pain transmission pathways" and prevents pain. In cluster headaches, the activity of certain parts of the brain changes. Oxygen restores the activity of these parts of the brain to normal, and its pain-relieving effect may be due to its direct effect on the brain.

## What is respiratory failure?

To understand this disease, you must first know the function of the lungs. When you breathe, air enters your body through your nose and mouth. This air then travels to the air sacs inside the lungs. These sacs are called alveoli.

Small blood vessels called capillaries are located in the walls of the air sac. When air reaches the alveoli, the oxygen in them travels through the walls into the blood flowing through the capillaries. At the same time, carbon dioxide travels from the capillaries to the alveoli. This process is called gas exchange. The disease can be acute (short-term) or chronic (continuous). Acute respiratory failure can develop rapidly and may require emergency treatment. But it starts slowly and lasts a long time.

Signs and symptoms of respiratory failure may include shortness of breath, rapid breathing, and starvation (such as when you cannot get enough oxygen). In severe cases, the signs and symptoms may include purple skin, lips and nails, dizziness, and drowsiness.

One of the main goals of treating respiratory failure is to transport oxygen to the lungs and other organs and remove carbon dioxide from the body. Another goal is to treat the root cause of the disease. Acute respiratory failure occurs when water collects in the air sacs of the lungs. When this condition occurs, the lungs cannot supply oxygen to the blood. Under these conditions, oxygen-rich blood will not reach the organs and their function will be impaired. Acute respiratory failure is also possible if the lungs are unable to excrete carbon dioxide into the blood.

Acute respiratory failure occurs when capillaries or small blood vessels around the air sacs cannot exchange carbon dioxide with oxygen. The disease can be acute or chronic. With acute respiratory failure, you will experience symptoms of hypoxia. In most cases, if left untreated, the disease can lead to death.


**Types and symptoms of acute respiratory failure**

Two types of acute and chronic respiratory failure; They are hypoxic and hypercapnia. Both types of disease can have serious side effects. Hypomaxia respiratory failure means that there is not enough oxygen in the blood, but blood carbon dioxide levels are almost normal. Hypercapnia respiratory failure means that the amount of carbon dioxide in the blood is very high, and the amount of oxygen in the blood is close to normal, or that there is not enough oxygen in the blood.

Acute respiratory symptoms depend on the cause and the level of carbon dioxide in the blood. People with high levels of carbon dioxide may have the following symptoms:

- ➢ Fast and steady breathing
- ➢ Confusion
- ➢ People with low blood oxygen levels may have the following symptoms:
- ➢ Inability to breathe
- ➢ The skin, fingers and lips turn blue

> Under these conditions, oxygen-rich blood does not reach the organs and their function will be impaired. Acute respiratory failure is also possible if the lungs are unable to excrete blood carbon dioxide.

> People with acute pulmonary insufficiency and low blood oxygen levels may have the following symptoms:

> Restlessness

> Anxiety

> Sleep Pollution

> Loss of consciousness

> Fast and shallow breathing

> Rapid heart rate

> Irregular heartbeat (arrhythmia)

> Excessive sweating

**What are the causes of respiratory failure?**

Diseases and conditions that interfere with breathing can cause respiratory failure. These disorders may affect the muscles, nerves, bones, or tissues that support breathing, or they may directly affect the lungs. When breathing is impaired, the lungs cannot easily carry oxygen to their blood and remove carbon dioxide from the blood (gas exchange). This disability can lower oxygen levels or increase carbon dioxide or both in the blood.

Respiratory failure can be caused by the following:

• Conditions that affect the nerves and muscles that control breathing. Examples of these causes include muscular dystrophy, amyotrophic lateral sclerosis (ALS), spinal cord injury, and stroke.

• Damage to the tissues and ribs around the lungs. Injury to the chest can cause this type of injury.

• Spine problems, such as scoliosis (curvature of the spine). This condition can affect the bones and muscles used to breathe.

• Excessive use of drugs or alcohol. Excessive consumption of these substances affects the area of the brain that controls breathing. In this condition, breathing becomes slow and shallow.

• Pulmonary diseases such as COPD, chronic obstructive pulmonary disease (pneumonia), ARDS, acute respiratory distress syndrome, pulmonary embolism, and cystic fibrosis. These diseases and conditions can affect the flow of air and blood in and out of the lungs. Of course, ARDS and pneumonia affect gas exchange in the alveoli.

• Acute lung injuries. For example, inhaling harmful fumes can damage the lungs. People with diseases or conditions that affect the muscles, nerves, bones, or tissues that support breathing are at risk for respiratory failure. People with lung disease are also at risk for respiratory failure.

**Treatment methods for respiratory failure**

Treatment of acute respiratory failure depends on its underlying cause. For example, respiratory failure due to scoliosis may require surgery to correct the spine so that the lungs and heart can function efficiently. A person with acute respiratory failure will usually need an extra source of oxygen. This may involve a form of mechanical artificial respiration in which a doctor inserts a plastic tube into a patient's throat. This provides the oxygen and pressure needed for the lungs to function more efficiently.

Physicians typically use this method of oxygenation as long as they can slow, eliminate, or reverse the underlying cause of acute respiratory failure. Other treatment strategies for acute respiratory failure include:

• Medications, such as antibiotics to treat infections and diuretics to reduce fluid in the lungs and body

• Swing or vibration of the chest wall to loosen the mucus in the lungs

• Sleep breathing, in which the person lies on their stomach and oxygen is supplied through an artificial respiration device.

• Extracorporeal membrane oxygenation, which includes the use of a cardiovascular bypass device to receive blood from the body and the supply of oxygen to reduce the working pressure on the heart and lungs.

Your doctor may prescribe medications to calm the patient that facilitate breathing with a ventilator. Because acute respiratory failure is a serious condition, treatment can be time consuming.

**Prevention of acute respiratory problems**

Not all causes of acute respiratory failure can be prevented. However, in the case of pneumonia and some other airway-related diseases, one can take steps to protect the lungs, including:

> Avoid smoking, which can damage the lungs
> See a doctor at the first sign of a bacterial infection such as fever, cough, and excessive mucus production
> Take all medications prescribed by your doctor to maintain heart and lung health
> If necessary, use assistive devices to maintain oxygen levels
> Adequate levels of physical activity to strengthen lung function

**Isolation of the patient from the ventilator**

Isolation of the patient from a mechanical ventilator or ventilator refers to the gradual cessation of supportive ventilation in patients whose large respiratory needs are met by spontaneous ventilation. In some patients this process is done quickly (less than or equal to 3 days) and in some patients, this process is longer than 3 days, so that sometimes the patient is separated from the mechanical ventilator for weeks or even months. it takes time.

Undoubtedly, determining the readiness of patients before starting the process of separation from the mechanical ventilation device is of great importance, and the greatest responsibility for determining the readiness of patients to separate from the mechanical ventilation device rests with nurses working in intensive care units. Nurses should look at the predictors of successful separation from a mechanical ventilator to determine if the patient can be removed from the mechanical ventilation system as soon as possible without any possible complications.

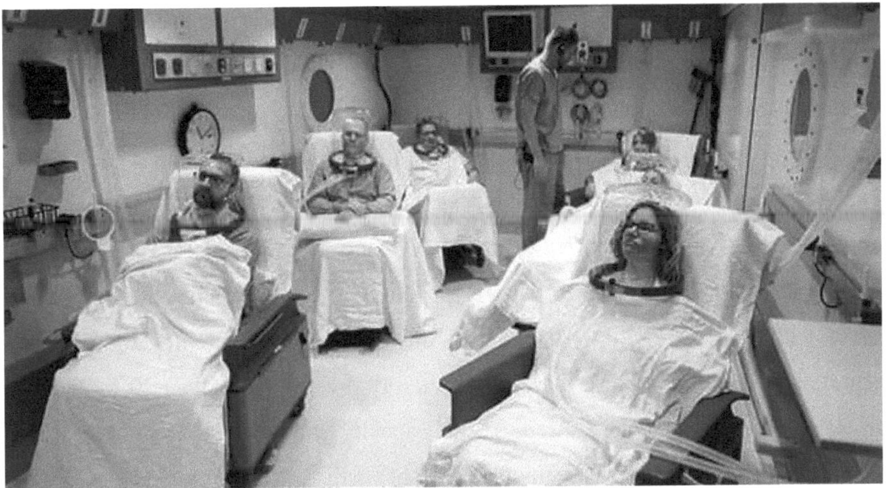

**Figure 13.** Hyperbaric oxygen therapy

Because there are no single predictors for separating patients from mechanical ventilation in medical and nursing books and articles. An attempt has been made to summarize the various theories of experts in this field. Separation from the mechanical ventilation device is the process of moving from the ventilation dependence to voluntary breathing, which should be followed immediately after placing the patient on the mechanical ventilation device to check the readiness of patients to separate from the mechanical ventilation device. Isolation of the patient from the mechanical ventilation system is influenced by factors such as the duration of mechanical ventilation, the physical condition of the patient's body such as respiratory muscle strength, the presence of underlying respiratory diseases, psychological dependence on the mechanical ventilation system, the presence of anxiety, malnutrition and immobility. Therefore, before starting the separation process, the patient's readiness to be separated from the mechanical ventilation device should be checked.

Readiness to isolate patients from mechanical ventilation is determined by ensuring physiological stability, hemodynamic stability, lung function, gas exchange status, spontaneous ventilation capacity, and patients' level of consciousness. Other indicators are mentioned as criteria for separation from mechanical ventilation, which include clinical status and objective measurements. In order to isolate the clinical condition from the mechanical ventilation device, the patient should be evaluated for effective cough preparation, absence of excessive secretions in the airway, improvement of underlying problems that cause his intubation.

Also, objective measurements include evaluation of patients in terms of clinical stability, stability of cardiovascular status (systolic pressure 90 to 160 mm Hg), stability of metabolic status, adequate oxygenation, arterial oxygen saturation (more than 90 with 40 fio2), PEEP (less than 8 cm of water), Adequate pulmonary function, respiration rate (less than 35), maximal expiratory pressure (less than 20 to 25 cm), current volume (greater than 5 ml / kg), vital capacity (greater than 10 ml / kg), RF to VT ratio less than 105 breaths per minute), lack of significant respiratory acidosis, state of consciousness and no need to take sedatives.

Separation of the patient from the ventilator or weaning is a process of movement from ventilation dependence to voluntary respiration. Isolation of the patient from the device to factors such as duration of ventilation, physical condition of the body such as body and strength of respiratory muscles, the presence of underlying respiratory diseases, psychological dependence on the ventilator, the presence of anxiety, malnutrition, immobility and. . . . it depends.


**Criteria for separating the patient from the ventilator**

I.  The patient can have 21% of $FiO_2$ and voluntary breathing, $PaO_2$ equal to or more than 60 mm Hg with an oxygen saturation of about 90% or more.

II.  All symptoms related to pathological processes should be controlled to stop the patient's fever. In the chest photo, the lungs should be clean. No dangerous dysrhythmia. The patient's hemodynamic status is constant.

III.  The patient is awake and has the ability to breathe spontaneously.

IV. The patient's normal airway is completely open.

V. In case of receiving oxygen with less than 5% and PEEP with 5 cm of water or less than PaO2 higher than 70 mm Hg.

VI. The current volume of the tail in the patient's spontaneous breathing is equal to or more than 5 kg / ml.

VII. The amount of ventilation per minute is more than 5 liters per minute and should not exceed 10 liters per minute.

VIII. The vital capacity of the patient is more than 10-15 kg / ml.

IX. The patient's tail pressure is equal to or more than 20 cm of water.

X. The patient's breathing rate is equal to or less than 25 breaths per minute.

XI. The amount of arterial blood gases is normal.

XII. The patient's circulatory status is stable and corrected.

XIII. The patient is able to discharge from his airways.

XIV. Static compliance is more than 25 cmH$_2$O / ml. At the time of separation from the device, the patient should be constantly monitored for symptoms such as shortness of breath, fatigue, anxiety, sweating, paleness or cyanosis, drowsiness, restlessness.

**Conditions for reconnecting the patient to the ventilator**

a. Systolic pressure decreases by 20 mm Hg or increases by more than 30 mm Hg.

b. The diastolic pressure varies by 10 mm or more.

c. The number of breaths reaches more than 25 to 30 breaths per minute. Increasing more than 10 breaths per minute and decreasing it to less than 8 breaths per minute indicates the patient's fatigue.

d. The pulse rate increases by more than 20 beats per minute or the heart rate reaches more than 125 beats per minute.

e. Frequent occurrence of premature ventricular contractions (PVC).

f. Breathing with a lot of effort and is tedious.

g. Severe abdominal paradox, which indicates insufficient diaphragmatic contraction and fatigue in the patient to continue voluntary breathing.

h.  Arterial blood gas (ABG) levels become abnormal.

**Successful separation of the patient from the ventilator**

> 12 to 24 hours before separation, the patient should have stable and acceptable blood pressure without the use of vasopressor drugs. Low doses of dopamine may be used to maintain renal perfusion.

> Low doses of intravenous TNG may be used to counteract the sudden increase in venous blood return due to relieving positive ventilatory pressure and to reduce cardiac pressure.

> S in general, CNS depressant drugs should be avoided. Broncho constrictors such as indral and neuromuscular blocking drugs and some antibiotics should also be avoided.

> Aminophylline may be used during separation, which can cause dilatation of the bronchi and increase the force of contraction of the diaphragm and heart muscle.

> Electrolyte imbalance, especially in patients with respiratory muscle atrophy due to prolonged artificial ventilation, can weaken the respiratory muscles.

> It is better for the patient to be sitting or semi-sitting when separating for better diaphragm activity.

> If there are defecation problems that can cause bloating and electrolyte disturbance, correct it.

**Methods of separating the ventilator from the patient**

How to use T Tube (T)?

CP - CPAP method

Si -SiMV method

PS pressure support method

After examining the patients' readiness for separation from the mechanical ventilation device and the positive indicators of successful separation from the ventilator, the patient should be separated. There are three main ways to separate a mechanical ventilator. These methods include the use of the T-piece and CPAP mode, the use of SIMV mode and the use of PSV mode. It should be noted that PSV mode is often used in combination with SIMV mode to reduce respiratory work in the patient.

Using the T-piece, the patient can be alternately separated from the mechanical ventilator to breathe spontaneously. To facilitate the patient's spontaneous breathing, it is removed from the device and a T-shaped tube is connected to the patient's tracheostomy tube or tracheal tube. One end of the T-tube is connected to the oxygen tank and the other end is free. In this case, the patient breathes without connecting to a mechanical ventilator and while using extra oxygen.

The T-piece is alternately removed and the patient is connected to a mechanical ventilator using CPAP mode. Gradually, by increasing the time of using the T-piece and decreasing the time of using the mechanical ventilation device with CPAP mode, the patient will reach a stage where he can use the T-piece for a longer period of time without the need for mechanical ventilation support. And have no respiratory fatigue.

In the method of using SIMV mode for isolation, the goal is to gradually reduce the number of forced breaths as the number of spontaneous breaths of the patient increases. So that in the end, the number of forced breaths of the mechanical air conditioner reaches zero and the patient has a sufficient number of spontaneous breaths.

It is used in PSV mode in patients with normal spontaneous respiration rate. It should be noted that these patients should have no respiratory distress and the current volume of their spontaneous breathing should be at the desired level (8-10 cc per kg). Gradually, the amount of pressure support is reduced during separation, and if the patient is able to breathe spontaneously and without respiratory distress without reducing the current volume, the reduction continues to a level of 3-5 cm of water. Here the patient can be completely Detached from mechanical ventilation.


**Symptoms of patient intolerance of mechanical ventilation**

If these signs and symptoms occur, the patient should be placed back on the mechanical ventilator.

**Respiratory signs and symptoms:** increase in the number of breaths to 30 to 35 times per minute, abnormal breathing pattern, paradoxical breathing, use of respiratory auxiliary muscles, expiratory flow volume less than 5 ml / kg, decrease in arterial oxygen saturation to less 85%, decrease or increase in $CO_2$, decrease in pao2 to less than 60 mm Hg.

**Hemodynamic changes:** changes in heart rate, angina, new dysrhythmias such as atrial fibrillation with rapid ventricular response, conduction disorders, changes in the ST segment, changes in blood pressure, changes in temperature and excessive sweating

**Neurological changes:** Anxiety, restlessness and drowsiness that can indicate hypoxia or hypercapnia.

In another study, indicators indicating failure in the separation process are divided into two categories of subjective and objective indicators. Mental symptoms include restlessness and anxiety, depressed mood, excessive sweating, cyanosis, evidence of increased effort, symptoms of respiratory distress (sweating and breathing with auxiliary muscles), and shortness of breath.

Objective indicators also include $pao_2$ (less than 60-50), fio2 more than 50% or arterial blood saturation less than 80 (paco2) more than 50 (PH) less than 32.7 (ratio of respiration to VT) more Out of 105 (number of breaths), more than 35 breaths per minute (FR), more than 140 beats per minute (systolic pressure), more than 180 mm Hg (or more than 20% increase in basal blood pressure).

Nurse responsibilities during separation:

I. The nurse should be familiar with separation modes and related goals.

II. The nurse should obtain the cooperation of the patient and his family in the separation process.

III. The nurse should begin the separation process during the hours of the day when medical, nursing, or respiratory support is available.

IV. The nurse should do things like dialysis, physiotherapy and... Avoid before or during separation.

V. The nurse should pay attention to the patient's position, whether he is half-sitting or fully seated.

VI. The nurse, if necessary, should perform intra-tracheal suctioning before placement to reduce the resistance of the airways.

VII. If necessary, the nurse should use bronchodilators.

VIII. The nurse should pay attention to the size of the endotracheal tube. It is 7 to 5.8 in women and 7.5 to 9 in men.

IX. The nurse should collect and record baseline information on vital signs, state of consciousness, heart rhythm, and pulse oximetry values before attempting to isolate or reduce ventilator support.

X. The nurse should examine the patient for signs and symptoms of excessive respiratory work that causes the patient to begin fatigue.

**Patient care under mechanical ventilation**

In order to provide nursing care to a patient admitted to the ICU ward, which is mechanically ventilated with a ventilator, first the various systems of the body must be carefully examined and finally the patient's problems and nursing diagnoses can be extracted.

**Examine the respiratory system**

➢ **Respiratory system examination:** For initial examination of the patient under ventilator, the chest should be observed for symmetrical breathing and the presence of abnormal breathing patterns. Lung sounds (bronchial and vesicular) in terms of symmetry, ventilation of both lungs, the presence of ral. After the hearing, if necessary, the patient should be sucked or, if possible, undergo respiratory physiotherapy. The patient's chest should be carefully touched for subcutaneous emphysema and its progression, especially in the presence of a tracheostomy or chest tube implantation and in rib fractures. The patient's lung image should be checked frequently for signs of improvement or regression. Also, the results of ABG test are of special importance for the patient in terms of adequacy of ventilation.

> **Examination of the endotracheal tube:** To ensure adequate ventilation of both lungs, the end of the tube should be at least three centimeters above the carina (where the trachea divides). After annotation, breathing sounds should be heard on both sides. If ventilation is appropriate, the exit of the tube from the mouth or nose should be marked with glue or magic to be informed of the displacement of the tube in subsequent inspections. To ensure proper placement of the tube, a lung photograph should be taken.

> **Examination of the tracheal tube cuff:** The filled cuff can cause pressure on the trachea, reduce blood flow to the area, and lead to damage to the tracheal wall and vocal cords. To prevent this complication, the cuff should be emptied for a few minutes every 2 hours after careful suction of the mouth and throat. Usually, the maximum pressure exerted by the inflated cuff should not exceed 15-20 mm Hg.

> **Examination of pulmonary secretions:** Because the patient is not able to cough effectively under a ventilator, pulmonary secretions should be performed if necessary.

> **Chest tube examination:** The patient should be checked for respiratory distress after implantation of the chest tube.

> Pneumothorax may be compressive due to malfunction of the tube, with symptoms of severe shortness of breath, paradoxical chest movements, dilation of the jugular veins, cyanosis, hypotension, shock, and chest hyperresonance as a whole.

- Observe the continuity of chest tube drainage
- Observe the movement of fluid in the tube with each breath, to check the function of the chest tube
- Control the amount, color and characteristics of the vessel every 5 minutes in the first minutes after intubation and then

every hour if the fluid is bloody and report in the vessel more than 150 ml per hour, which can be due to the presence of a foci Bleeding is active in the area.

> **Checking the correct ventilator setting**: The adjuster and ventilator should be checked with what is written on the cardex and the chart above the patient's head. All parameters of the device including: Peep-Mode-RR-VT-Fio2 must be carefully adjusted and recorded in the patient chart by mentioning the time.

## Check the circulatory system

**Pulse:** The patient's pulse should be controlled in terms of number, order, quality and strength. Remember that in the ICU, routine control of the radial pulse alone is not enough, but due to the patient's immobility and the possibility of thrombosis and vascular problems, foot pulses such as Dorsey Pedis to be controlled and recorded on both feet in each shift.

**Blood pressure:** It is very important to control systolic and diastolic blood pressure and then calculate the pulse pressure. Pulse pressure is the difference between systolic and diastolic pressures: PP = S - D. Normally, for example, at a blood pressure of 120/80, the pulse pressure is equal to 40 mm Hg

Observation of dilation of cervical veins: To evaluate the incidence of heart failure in patients who are under ventilator for a long time.

**CVP control:** CVP control is required every hour. Its normal value is between +4 and +10 cm of water and indicates the return of venous blood.

**Pulmonary capillary wedge pressure control:** should be monitored every hour. Its normal level is between 6- and 12-mm Hg. If the amount of 18 mm Hg increases, it indicates pulmonary congestion. And when its level reaches more than 25 to 30 mm Hg, it indicates the occurrence of pulmonary edema.

**Controlling the filling time of capillaries under the nail:** To do this, you should press the patient's fingernail with your finger for about 5 seconds, then lift your finger immediately and start counting the numbers in seconds until the pink color of the nail returns. Normally, this time is less than 2 seconds. Between 2 and 3 seconds indicates a blood pump failure and more than that indicates the patient shows symptoms of shock.

**Cardiac hearing:** The heart should be audited for the presence of a third sound (gallop S3) which is one of the first signs of heart failure in the patient.

**Evaluation of the patient's level of relaxation and anxiety:** Factors that cause sudden and severe anxiety and anxiety in the patient under mechanical ventilation are: decreased oxygenation, pain and fear. Therefore, if the patient suddenly develops such conditions, he should first be examined for the amount of oxygen received, the need for suction and proper ventilation. Then, according to the patient's non-verbal communication and touch of his body, he examined the amount of pain in his body. Keep in mind that most mechanically ventilated patients experience pain and fatigue in the back and pressure areas due to immobility and need to change position and massage the affected areas. Verbal communication, eye contact, and touching the patient during nursing care or whenever the patient needs them can significantly reduce the patient's fear and anxiety.

**Assess the level of consciousness based on the Glasgow GCS rating criteria**
The state of consciousness and its progression or regression during ventilator treatment should be considered by intensive care unit nurses. Decreasing GCS increases their mortality. Patients with a GCS score of less than 5 have a mortality rate of about 50%.

**Organ Examination: Examination of the patient's organs is important for edema, phlebitis cyanosis, heat and humidity.**

**Urinary tract examination**

- ➢ Checking this system should be done every hour as follows:
- ➢ Calculate the amount of fluid received per hour
- ➢ Calculate the amount of fluid excreted per hour
- ➢ Comparison of fluid absorption and excretion
- ➢ Examination of the catheter entry area for inflammation and infection
- ➢ Check the characteristics of urine
- ➢ Examination of the digestive system

Patients under ventilator may be NPOs or receive high-calorie, high-protein fluids through a gastric tube, jejunostomy, or ileostomy. Hyperfusion may also be used in patients with a negative nitrogen balance.

**Respiratory physiotherapy, and heart surgery**

Physiotherapy in respiratory patients includes correcting the respiratory pattern, strengthening the muscles of the respiratory system, draining the secretions into the lungs and airways, as well as stimulating cough reflux and teaching breathing techniques and breathing exercises.

Respiratory physiotherapy after heart surgery includes two types of breathing in the form of abdominal breathing and rib breathing and effective and strong coughing. To do abdominal breathing, the patient lies on a bed, puts his hand on his abdomen, and takes a deep breath so that the hand moves upward on the abdomen. Pause for a moment and let the air out of your lungs.

Objectives of the patient's physiotherapy in the cardiac surgery department

i. Improving blood circulation in the limbs by doing active sports movements

ii. Training and performing breathing exercises to improve the respiratory condition and discharge of secretions

iii. Prevention of possible atelectasis

iv. Encouraging the patient to general mobility of the body and starting the patient as soon as possible after surgery

v. Teaching how to make effective coughs and body.

**Work factor: Nurse and physiotherapist**

1. Explain heart surgery to the patient in simple language.
2. Familiarize the patient with the tubes connected to his body after the operation, such as urinary catheter, NGT, Drain, Chest tube, endotracheal tube, etc.
3. Assess respiratory status, pulmonary secretion rate, accumulation of pulmonary secretions, and abnormal lung sounds.
4. Teach the patient breathing exercises, limb exercises, and how to cough painlessly.
5. Do active limb exercises.
6. Practice breathing exercises with the patient in order to learn and do it properly after the operation.
7. Introduce the patient to a spirometer and explain how to practice properly with it after the operation.
8. Practice effective and painless coughing with the patient.
9. Record your findings and actions.

**Gear breathing**

The patient lies on the bed as before and this time puts his hands on the chest under the breasts and tries to enter as much air as possible into the lungs with a deep breath so that the ribs open under his hands. After a moment, the pause expels air from the lungs. Breathe in this way several times, then place your hand on top of your breasts, and this time try to expand your upper chest with deep breaths. (Of course, it is better for the patient to raise the back of the bed a little and put a pillow under his knees before doing these exercises.)

**Strong and effective cough training**

The patient sits on the bed, grabs a pillow and presses it to his chest, then tries to cough hard and effectively. (Gets the opposite shoulder with his hand.)

Do it carefully as instruct by your physiotherapist. These procedures are performed ten times a day, three times a day:

1. Lie on the bed and bend and straighten your ankles.
2. Rotate your ankles left and right.
3. Bend and straighten your knees in turn.
4. Move your legs up in turns with a straight knee.
5. Move your shoulders up.
6. Fist your hands together and move both hands up and down together.

**How to get out of bed:** First, turn your whole body to the left or right side, then press the elbow of the lower hand on the bed and try to get up from the bed and sit down. Pause for a moment, then place your hands on your knees and stand with a little pressure on your knees.

1- Never take a deep breath or cough in a row and fast because it may cause fatigue or dizziness.
2- When standing and walking, you should keep your back and chest straight and straight. You should not be hunchbacked.
3- After leaving the ICU and entering the surgery ward, start walking with the doctor's permission and try to walk more day by day.
4- If you have any questions or problems, ask the staff of the department for help.
5- When resting on the bed, you should change your position every two hours.
6- When changing position or exercising, be careful of the wires and tubes connected to your body and inform the ward nurses about unusual discharges.
7- After discharge from the hospital, do the exercises prescribed for you by your physiotherapist on a daily basis.
8- Try to walk at least half an hour a day.
9- Do not do heavy work for at least two months.

**How to use the spromometer?**

When lying on the bed, raise the back of the bed, then take the spirometer tube with one hand and put it in your mouth, and with the other hand, hold the spirometer and hold it in front of your face so that the ball moves inside the device with each Watch the tail move up and down. Then take a deep breath and try to move the ball inside the device and raise it to the size prescribed for you and hold it in front of the desired number for a few seconds, then slowly exhale the air out of the lungs. Hold this again in front of the desired number, then gently blow air out of the lungs and repeat. If you feel tired after working with the machine several times, stop your training and start training again after a while.

**Duration and frequency of work with spirometer**

• **The day before surgery:** The patient should work with the device regularly to fully learn how to use it properly.

• **The first and second day after surgery:** When waking up, exercise every two hours until fatigue.

• **Third day after surgery:** Practice with the machine every one to two hours.

• **Fourth day after surgery:** Practice with the machine every four hours.

**The need for cardiac physiotherapy**

High mortality from heart disease has prompted specialists to look at the physiotherapy capabilities of the field of physiotherapy, thereby reducing a significant amount of complications and pain before and after heart surgery. The high rate of deaths due to cardiovascular diseases in our country made us talk more about the importance of cardiac physiotherapy.

Some of Dr. Shirvi's experiences indicate that cardiac rehabilitation is one of the most important sub-disciplines of physiotherapy and says: Rehabilitation of the patient's cardiopulmonary system and locomotor system following open heart surgery to prevent mortality, recurrence and progression The level of physical and mental health of the patient plays an important role. In open heart surgery, the nourishing arteries of the heart tissue (coronary arteries) that are severely clogged and unable to fully oxygenate the cells of the heart tissue, with healthy arteries taken from other parts of the body, especially arteries.

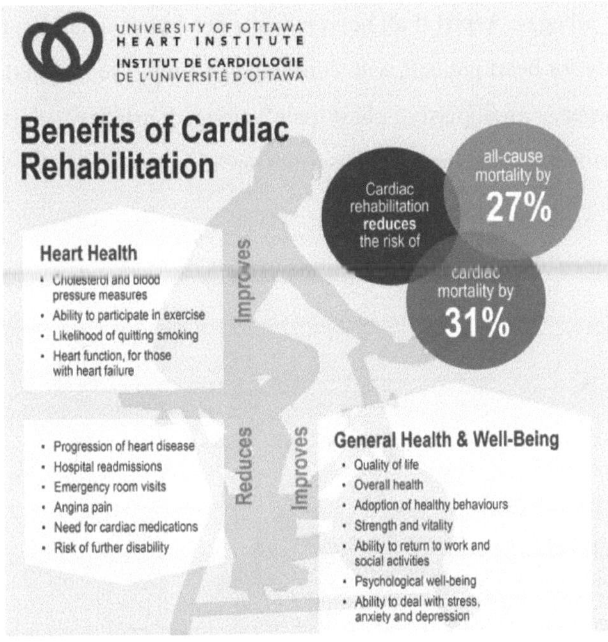



**Figure 14.** Cardiac PreHab Aims to Better Prepare Patients for Surgery

The legs are replaced. After reconstructive surgery, the establishment of normal blood flow in these arteries guarantees the success of the operation and the patient's return to normal life, which is addressed in cardiac rehabilitation using various methods.

Perform effective and complete breathing, prevent the accumulation of secretions in the lungs following anesthesia and hospitalization, chest mobility with a wide line of operation in front of the chest, reduce pain in the operation area and ribs, get out of bed as soon as possible and move independently and control limb inflammation in particular, lower extremity surgery is one of the important goals of cardiac physiotherapy.

In the past, doctors, especially patients, thought that cardiac rehabilitation and therapeutic exercises in the postoperative period are associated with serious risks and may not have much effect on improving the patient's health, but today with the advancement of physiotherapy and careful monitoring and control of conditions Patient during treatment, this method is used completely safely in many cardiovascular diseases and at all ages. Asked if all heart patients need physiotherapy, he said: "This treatment is only for heart patients with coronary artery disease (angina), heart attack, open heart surgery, angioplasty, chest pain, clogged arteries." Peripheral, heart transplant, heart failure, and heart valve surgery are effective.

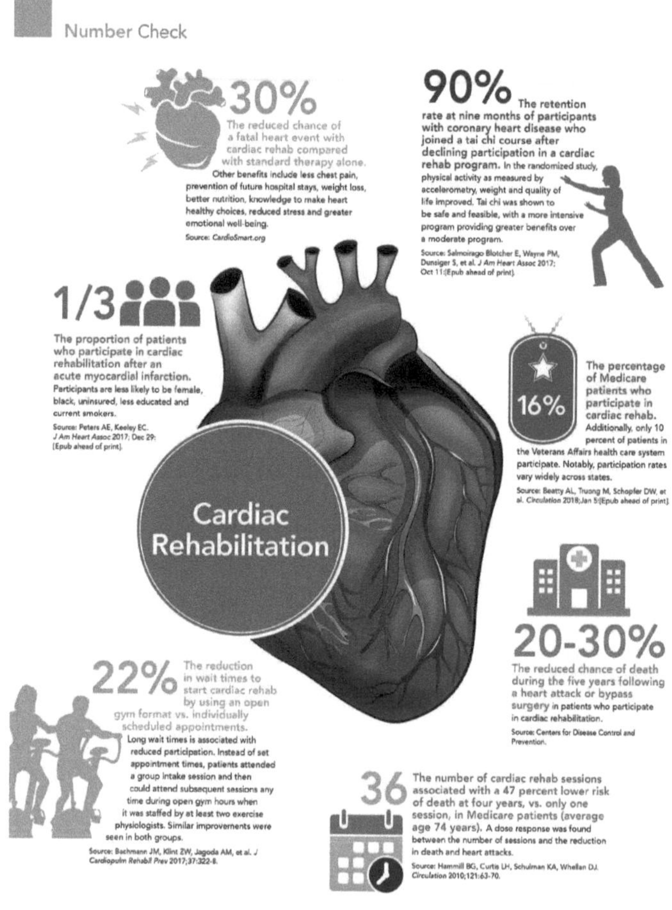


**Figure 15.** Number Check

This treatment reduces the risk of death from heart disease by 15 to 25 percent, as well as improves quality of life, increases smoking cessation, weight loss, lowers blood lipids, reduces depression and increases the patient's functional level.

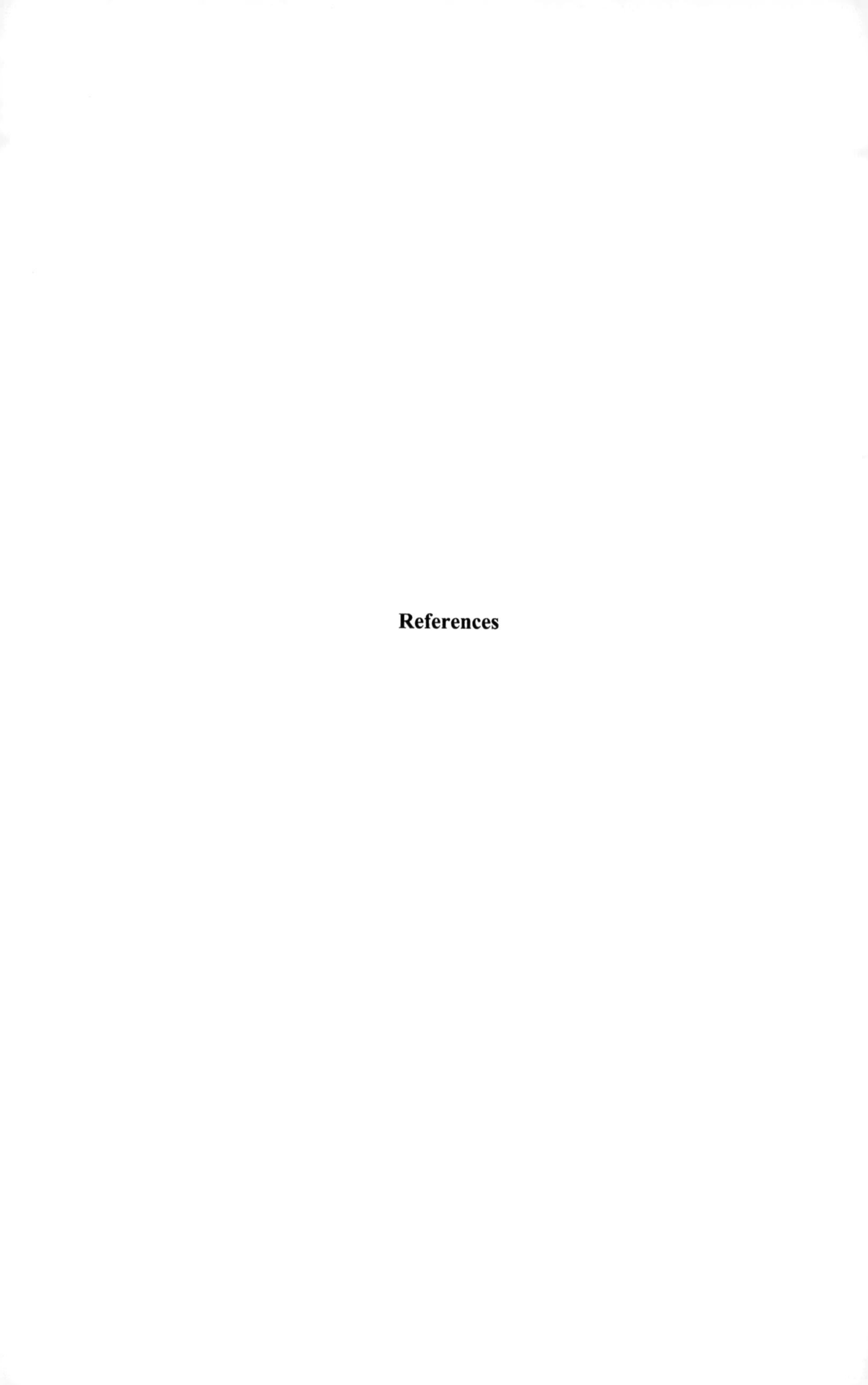

**References**

Bolster D, Manias E. Person-centered interactions between nurses and patients during medication activities in an acute hospital setting: qualitative observation and interview study. Int J Nurs Stud. 2010 Feb; 47 (2): 154-65.

Thorne SE, Harris SR, Mahoney K, Con A, McGuinness L. The context of health care communication in chronic illness. Patient Educ Couns. 2004 Sep; 54 (3): 299-306.

Potter. Patricia Ann. Principles and techniques of nursing Potter and Perry. Translated by Susan Oveysi and ... First. Healthy. Tehran 1387

Taylor. Carol, Taylor Principles of Nursing. Concepts of partial nursing. Translation of Afsaneh Eftekhari Mansouravel .Bashri. Tehran 1391

Lindberg JB, Hunter ML, Kruszewski AZ. Introduction to nursing: concepts, issues and opportunities. 2nd ed. Philadelphia: J.B. Lippincott Company; 1994.

Aein F, Alhani F, Mohammadi E, Kazemnejad A. [Marginating the interpersonal relationship: Nurses and parent's experiences of communication in pediatric wards]. Iranian Journal of Nursing Research. 2008; 3 (8.9): 71-83. (Persian)

Mohammadzadeh Sh, Bakhtiari S, Moshtagh Z, Ebrahimi E. [Communication barriers from nurses' and elderly patint's points of views at medical-surgical wards]. Journal of Nursing & Midwifery,

Special HS, Carpenter DR. Qualitative research in nursing: Advancing the humanistic imperative. Philadelphia: Lippincott Williams & Wilkins; 2007.

Krippendorff KH. Content analysis: An introductory to its methodology. 2nd ed. California: Sage Publication, Inc; 2004

Graneheim UH, Lundman B. Qualitative content analysis in nursing research: concepts, procedures and measures to achieve trustworthiness. Nurse Educ Today. 2004 Feb; 24 (2): 105-12.

Fakhr-Movahedi A, Salsali M, Negharandeh R, Rahnavard Z. A qualitative content analysis of nurse-patient communication in Iranian nursing. Int Nurs Rev. 2011 Jun; 58 (2): 171-80.

Caris-Verhallen WM, de Gruijter IM, Kerkstra A, Bensing JM. Factors related to nurse communication with elderly people. J Adv Nurs. 1999 Nov; 30 (5): 1106-17.

Magnus VS, Turkington L. Communication interaction in ICU - Patient and staff experiences and perceptions. Intensive Crit Care Nurs. 2006 Jun; 22 (3): 167-80.

Anoosheh M, Zarkhah S, Faghihzadeh S, Vaismoradi M. Nurse-patient communication barriers in Iranian nursing. Int Nurs Rev. 2009 Jun; 56 (2): 243-9.

Baillie L. An exploration of nurse-patient relationships in accident and emergency. Accid Emerg Nurs. 2005 Jan; 13 (1): 9-14

Rana D, Upton D. Psychology for nurses. Harlow: pearson Higher education; 2009.

Hagerty BM, Patusky KL. Reconceptualizing the nurse-patient relationship. J Nurs Scholarsh. 2003; 35 (2): 145-50.

Shattell M. Nurse-patient interaction: a review of the literature. J Clin Nurs. 2004 Sep; 13 (6): 714- 22

Suikkala A, Leino-Kilpi H, Katajisto J. Factors related to the nursing student-patient relationship: the students' perspective. Nurse Educ Today. 2008 Jul; 28 (5): 539-49.

Pytel C, Fielden NM, Meyer KH, Albert N. Nurse-patient / visitor communication in the emergency department. J Emerg Nurs. 2009 Sep; 35 (5): 406-11.

Mottram A. Therapeutic relationships in day surgery: a grounded theory study. J Clin Nurs. 2009 Oct; 18 (20): 2830-7.

Finch LP. Patients' communication with nurses: Relational communication and preferred nurse behaviors. International Journal of Human Caring. 2006; 10 (4): 14-22.

Chiovitti RF. Nurses' meaning of caring with patients in acute psychiatric hospital settings: a grounded theory study. Int J Nurs Stud. 2008 Feb; 45 (2): 203-23.

Allen D. The nursing-medical boundary: A negotiated order? Sociology of Health & Illness. 1997 Sep; 19 (4): 498-520.

Takrouri MSM, Intensive care unit. The Internet Journal of Health, 2004; 3 (2)

Meleis AI. Theoretical nursing: Development and progress. 3rd ed. Philadelphia: Lippincott Williams & Wilkins; 2005.

Taylor M., Odell M., Nursing care for critically ill patient. The intensive care society, 2011; 12 (1); 10

Nurses Association of New Brunswick. Standard for the therapeutic nurse-client relationship. Available at: http://www.nanb.nb.ca/ Accessed, 2000.

McDonald DD, Laporta M, Meadows-Oliver M. Nurses' response to pain communication from patients: a post-test experimental study. Int J Nurs Stud. 2007 Jan; 44 (1): 29-35.

College of Nurses of Ontario. Practice standards: Therapeutic nurse-client relationship. Available at: http://www.cno.org/ Accessed, 2004.

Ito M, Lambert VA. Communication effectiveness of nurses working in a variety of settings within one large university teaching hospital in western Japan. Nurs Health Sci. 2002 Dec; 4 (4): 149-53.

Gurses A P., Carayon P., Performance obstacle of intensive care nurses. Nursing research, 2007; 56 (3); 185-194

Abbey M P., Understanding the work of intensive care nurses; a time and motion study. Thesis of master degree, School of nursing and midwifery, Griffith University, 2008

Scanlon A. Psychiatric nurses' perceptions of the constituents of the therapeutic relationship: a grounded theory study. J Psychiatr Ment Health Nurs. 2006 Jun; 13 (3): 319-29

Hosseini, M. M., Principles of Nursing Services Management. Tehran: Bashari Publications, 2008, first edition

Bowles N, Mackintosh C, Torn A. Nurses' communication skills: an evaluation of the impact of solution-focused communication training. J Adv Nurs. 2001 Nov; 36 (3): 347-54.

Yaghoubian, M., Nursing and Midwifery Management, Tehran: Bashari Publications, 1997, first edition

Aghabarary M, Mohammadi E, Varvani-Farahani A. Barriers to Application of Communicative Skills by Nurses in Nurse-Patient Interaction: Nurses and Patients' Perspective. Iran J Med Educ. 2009; 22 (61): 19-31. Persian.

McCabe C. Nurse-patient communication: an exploration of patients' experiences. J Clin Nurs. 2004 Jan; 13 (1): 41-9.

Abedi H, Alavi M, Aseman rafat N, Yazdani M. [Nurse-elderly patient's relationship experiences in hospital wards- a qualitative study]. Iranian Journal of Nursing and Midwifery Research. 2005; 5 (29): 5-16. (Persian)

Stephen P. Robbins. Translated by Dr. Ali Parsaian and Dr. Seyed Mohammad Aarabi. Fundamentals of Organizational Behavior: Cultural Research Office 2015

That Harvey and Christian Sanders and David Dixon. Social skills in interpersonal communication. Translated by Mehrdad Firooz Bakht-Khashayar Beigi. Third. Rash. Tehran. 2008

Instructions for submitting medical records and information, Ministry of Health and Medical Education, Deputy of Treatment, Office of Hospital Management and Clinical Services Excellence, Code of National Instruction A-P-7-3-35-1695

Dogas.Borley Witter. Principles of patient care..Volume one. Translated by Forouzan Atashzadeh. Shorideh and ... Golban. Tehran 2012

-Satisfaction. Mehdi, Stress Management, Ghaemieh Computer Research Center, Isfahan, Digital Publishing, 2012

Sharaf Din. Farzaneh, Job Stress and its Stress Management Ghaemieh Computer Research Center, Isfahan, Digital Publishing, 2012

Shidfar, Mohammad Reza Comprehensive book of public health. Volume one, second edition of the Ministry of Health, Medical Education / Deputy of Research and Technology.2010

Faizi, A., Abdi, M., Ansari, M., Mortality rate and its effective factors in patients admitted to intensive care units. Journal of Ardabil University of Medical Sciences, Volume 8, Number 4, Winter 2008, pp: 423-420

Masoudi Asl. Yerevan, Principles of Nursing Services Management, Second Edition, Jame Negar Publisher, 2016

Mirzakhani, Maryam and Davoodi, Alireza, 2019, Evaluation of MDR causes in patients connected to ventilator in ICU wards of Mazandaran Heart Center, 9th Specialized Congress on Infection Control and Sterilization, Medical Materials and Equipment, Tehran, https://civilica.com / doc / 998495

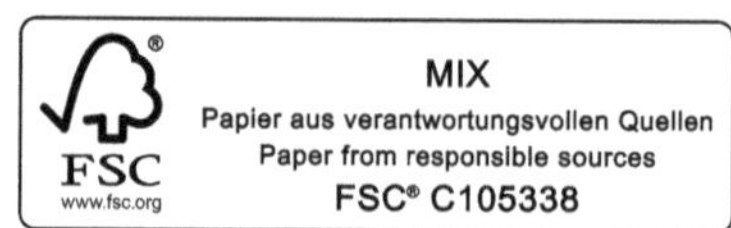

Printed by Books on Demand GmbH, Norderstedt / Germany